Atheroma to Heart Failure: A continuum of disease?

Atheroma to Heart Failure: A Continuum of Disease?

Edited by

Robert H. Anderson
Joseph Levy Professor in Paediatric Cardiac Morphology, National Heart and Lung Institute, London, UK

and

Philip A. Poole-Wilson
Simon Marks Professor of Cardiology, National Heart and Lung Institute, London, UK

Magdi H. Yacoub
Professor of Cardiothoracic Surgery, National Heart and Lung Institute, London, UK

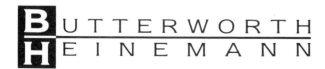

Butterworth-Heinemann Ltd
Linacre House, Jordan Hill, Oxford OX2 8DP

 PART OF REED INTERNATIONAL BOOKS

OXFORD LONDON BOSTON
MUNICH NEW DELHI SINGAPORE SYDNEY
TOKYO TORONTO WELLINGTON

First published 1991

British Library Cataloguing in Publication Data
Anderson, Robert H.
    Atheroma to heart failure: a continuum of disease?
    I. Title   II. Poole-Wilson, Philip A.
    III. Yacoub, Magdi H.
    616.1

ISBN 0 7506 1335 1

Library of Congress Cataloguing in Publication Data
Atheroma to heart failure: a continuum of disease?/edited by
    Robert H. Anderson and Philip A. Poole-Wilson.
        p.   cm. — (Royal Brompton series)
    Includes bibliographical references and index.
    ISBN 0 7506 1335 1:
    1. Heart—Diseases.   2. Heart—Pathophysiology.
        I. Anderson, Robert Henry.   II. Poole-Wilson,
        Philip A.   III. Yacoub, Magdi H.   IV. Series.
    [DNLM: 1. Heart Diseases. WG 200 C2675]
    RC681.C177   1991
    616.12—dc20
    DNLM/DLC   90-15179

Typeset by Latimer Trend and Co Ltd, Plymouth, Devon
Printed and bound by Hartnolls Ltd, Bodmin, Cornwall

Preface to the Series

Shortly after the end of the Second World World War, separate Institutes for Postgraduate Education were established as part of the University of London to encourage research into diseases of the chest and of the heart. Each Institute was associated with well-established Hospitals – the Institute for Diseases of the Chest with the Brompton and London Chest Hospitals, and the Institute of Cardiology with the National Heart Hospital.

Although these various Institutes and Hospitals were scattered throughout London, certain farsighted physicians noted the advantages to be gained by unifying their efforts. In the 1960s, therefore, the Institutes joined together as the Cardiothoracic Institute, while the Hospitals also adopted a central administration. The sites themselves, however, remained separate, although plans were established to bring them together. Within the last two years, these plans have finally come to fruition.

In 1988, the Lord Flowers, Vice-Chancellor of the University of London, opened the new premises of the Institute, which was renamed the National Heart and Lung Institute. In February, 1991, her Majesty the Queen opened the Sydney Street Wing of the new Royal Brompton National Heart and Lung Hospital, while the London Chest Hospital, still separate, was renamed the Victoria Park branch of the Hospitals.

We believe that these amalgamations now give us the opportunity to realize the potential envisaged by our predecessors when they proposed our union. They bring together cardiologists, chest physicians, surgeons, paediatricians, research workers, and all their associated specialities, on one site: a site with considerable potential for still further expansion. Already, since the Institute has been united on one site, it has become associated with the Thrombosis Research Institute and the Wynn Institute for Metabolic Research. Taken together, these combinations make us the largest postgraduate organization dedicated exclusively to diseases of the heart and lungs within Europe. As such, we believe we have need of a forum in which to discuss and disseminate the major researches and advances being made by our staff and their collaborators throughout the world. Thanks to the enthusiastic support of Butterworth-Heinemann, this will now be possible through the *Royal Brompton Reviews*.

It is our intention to produce two series of these reviews, one concerned with diseases of the heart and the other with diseases of the lung. This, the first review, is devoted to the patterns of disease occurring in the continuum which extends from coronary arterial atherosclerosis, through ischaemic heart disease, to heart failure. So as to ensure that these reviews maintain the standards expected from peer-reviewed material, we, as editors, have assembled an advisory board of internationally acknowledged experts in the fields of cardiology and cardiac surgery. We were delighted that all those we asked to join our board accepted. We hope that they will help us to maintain the high standard which we judge to have been achieved in this initial volume. It is our intention that the next review will address a topic concerned with disease of the lungs, and will be monitored and directed by our equally committed colleagues in thoracic medicine, who have assembled their own Board of experts.

In short, we anticipate that this will be the first of a series of *Royal Brompton Reviews* concerned with diseases of the heart and lungs.

Robert H. Anderson
Philip A. Poole-Wilson
Magdi H. Yacoub

Preface

This first volume of the *Royal Brompton Reviews* is a testament to the increasingly symbiotic relationship which is developing between academics and the pharmaceutical industry. The book would not have been possible without the enthusiastic support of Squibb Pharmaceuticals, now a part of Bristol Myers Squibb. The concept of a symposium to discuss the spectrum of disease from coronary atherosclerosis to terminal heart failure, and the options for treatment along the continuum, was first mooted by Dr David Blowers, and was supported thereafter by Dr Pam Lewis and Tim Bradley. Without their continuing support, the concept would have come to nothing. With their encouragement, we were able to gather both a distinguished faculty and an enthusiastic audience to discuss this topic at the National Heart and Lung Institute. With suitable cajoling, virtually all the contributors at our meeting agreed to expand and supplement their presentations to provide the chapters within our review. Equally distinguished colleagues stepped in to fill the small gaps judged to have been left in our initial programme.

We have taken care to edit these chapters to the best of our ability so as to provide a uniform overview of the patterns of disease which spring from our chosen continuum of disease. Our attempts to achieve uniformity were not always easy. We are still not sure whether all our authors are convinced that 'ischaemic heart disease' is a better term than 'coronary heart disease', and other readers may, therefore, be surprised to find scant mention of coronary heart disease in a volume concerned with coronary atherosclerosis. In terms of syntax, however, it can be argued that 'coronary heart disease' is a tautology, since, in medical terminology, 'coronary' as an adjective is only applied to the heart. It is also the case that ischaemic heart disease is, almost always, the consequence of coronary arterial disease.

To our mind, therefore, 'ischaemic heart disease' is at least as accurate a term as 'coronary heart disease', and much more grammatically appropriate! For this reason, it has been used throughout the volume to describe the process which others may still prefer to call 'coronary heart disease'. Apart from this discussion, and a brief mention in Chapter 2, the latter phrase will not be found within the review. The coverage of the process of disease, however, irrespective of the terms used for its description, is extensive and, we believe, authoritative.

The chapters of our review extend from an impassioned plea for early diagnosis of the atherosclerotic process by means of magnetic resonance; through discussions of the atherosclerotic plaque and its relationship to thrombosis, to transplantation of the heart for terminal failure, incorporating important advances in basic science related to the myocardial cell and the endothelium.

As editors, with our obvious bias, we are delighted with the scientific content of our first *Royal Brompton Review*. We hope the volumes which follow will be equally apposite.

Robert H. Anderson
Philip A. Poole-Wilson
Magdi H. Yacoub

Contributors

N.R. Banner
Harefield Hospital, Harefield, Middlesex, UK

P. Collins
Senior Lecturer and Honorary Consultant Cardiologist, National Heart and Lung Institute and Royal Brompton National Heart and Lung Hospitals, London

L. Dalla Libera
CNR Centre for Muscle Biology and Pathophysiology, Padova, Italy

C. Dal Palŭ
Clinica Medica I, University of Padova, Italy

M.J. Davies, MD, FRCPath, FACC
Department of Cardiovascular Pathology,
St George's Hospital Medical School, University of London

M.A. de Belder, MD, MRCP
Senior Registrar in Cardiology, Royal Brompton National Heart and Lung Hospitals, London

K. Fox
Consultant Cardiologist, Royal Brompton National Heart and Lung Hospitals, London

D. Hackett, MD, MRCP(I)
Cardiovascular Research Unit, Department of Medicine, Royal Postgraduate Medical School, Hammersmith Hospital, London

S.E. Harding
Lecturer in Cardiology, National Heart and Lung Institute, London

D. Longmore
Magnetic Resonance Unit,
Royal Brompton National Heart and Lung Hospitals, London; National Heart and Lung Institute, London

J.M. Mann
Department of Cardiovascular Pathology,
St George's Hospital Medical School,
University of London

D. Mulcahy
Senior Registrar in Cardiology, Royal Brompton National Heart and Lung
Hospitals, London

M.F. Oliver
Wynn Institute for Metabolic Research, National Heart and Lung Institute,
London

P. Pauletto
Clinica Medica I, University of Padova, Italy

A.C. Pessina
Clinica Medica I, University of Padova, Italy

P.A. Poole-Wilson
Professor of Cardiology,
National Heart and Lung Institute, London

E. Rowland
National Heart and Lung Institute, London; Royal Brompton National Heart and
Lung Hospitals, London

G. Scannapieco
Clinica Medica I, University of Padova, Italy

U. Sigwart
Consultant Cardiologist, Royal Brompton National Heart and Lung Hospitals,
London

S.R. Underwood
Marcus Sieff Senior Lecturer in Cardiac Imaging, National Heart and Lung
Institute, London

G. Vescovo
Clinica Medica I, University of Padova, Italy

M. Williams
Research Fellow, Royal Brompton National Heart and Lung Hospitals, London

M. Yacoub
Department of Cardiothoracic Surgery, National Heart and Lung Institute, London

Advisory Board

Contents

1

The natural history of ischaemic heart disease: is there a continuum?

Philip A. Poole-Wilson

In the UK, with a population of 56 million, 35 000 persons under the age of 65 years die each year of ischaemic heart disease, 200 000 sustain an acute myocardial infarction and 2 000 000 suffer from angina. These figures are not greatly different in many Western countries. The key question addressed in this volume is whether or not there is a continuum of heart disease extending from the early development of atheroma in the coronary arteries, through a thrombotic tendency to acute myocardial infarction and to heart failure. The issue is critical to doctors and health administrators trying to alleviate the sequels of heart disease in the general population.

The epidemiology of ischaemic heart disease is well established, and a number of risk factors have been identified. Over 50% of persons who will, in the following few years, develop acute myocardial infarction in the United Kingdom, can be predicted by a history of angina, a family history of ischaemic heart disease, smoking habit, the presence of diabetes and a raised blood pressure. The measurement of the concentration of cholesterol in the blood adds little further discriminatory information. Although that is encouraging, there still remains a sizeable group of patients who are admitted to hospital with acute myocardial infarction for whom there is, at present, no satisfactory explanation.

Atheroma in the coronary arteries becomes manifest as angina pectoris, sudden death or acute myocardial infarction. Sudden death is attributable to episodes of ventricular fibrillation, or to ventricular tachycardia degenerating into fibrillation. Whether this lethal event is an opportunistic arrhythmia dependent on chance circumstances and the substrate of fibrosis resulting from myocardial ischaemia, or whether the arrhythmia is the consequence of a transient, and possibly small, area of acute ischaemia in the myocardium is entirely unknown. The problem is that most information relates to those patients who come to medical attention because of recurrent ventricular tachycardia or who have been resuscitated from a cardiac arrest. A population study is needed.

Acute myocardial infarction carries a mortality of 10% during the period of hospitalization. A further 10% die in the following year, and the subsequent mortality is approximately 4% per year. The major causes of death (in 70%) in the acute episode are pulmonary oedema, circulatory collapse (both forms of heart failure), cardiac rupture or asystole. Later deaths may occur due to an arrhythmia, reinfarction, or heart failure.

Recent interest has been channelled in three directions: the identification of additional factors predicting the occurrence of infarction; the use of thrombolytic agents (or angioplasty) to open up the occluded coronary artery; and the limitation of damage to the infarcted heart. Following acute myocardial infarction, the damaged tissue forms a scar over a period of several weeks. The edge of the infarct may be clearly delineated to the naked eye but, under the microscope, peninsulas of damaged myocardium extend into the healthy tissue. The endocardium is commonly more extensively fibrotic than the epicardium. The entire healing process may be influenced by whether the artery supplying the area of infarction remains occluded or is reopened, either spontaneously or by treatment with thrombolytic agents. During the period of repair the heart must continue to provide the cardiac output.

This is achieved partly by the remaining myocardium contracting more strongly, and partly by the heart enlarging and changing its shape. Although this may be advantageous in the short term, in the longer term the size of the heart is a strong predictor of mortality. The enlargement of the heart occurs due to cell slippage in healthy myocardium and to cell slippage and stretching of fibrous tissue in the infarcted tissue. The distribution of fibrosis in the heart, stretch of cells, cell slippage, and alteration of myocardial geometry may all contribute not only to the occurrence of arrhythmias but also to the later development of heart failure. The possibility exists that prevention of this 'remodelling' of the heart may be beneficial.

The importance of such a scenario to those concerned with health provision, and the public at large, would depend on how often this 'continuum' from atheroma to heart failure occurs in the whole population. Figure 1.1 illustrates the problem. Heart failure may be a progressive condition where the function of the heart deteriorates with time due to increased stress in the wall of the heart itself and to changes in the peripheral circulation. Alternatively, the progression of heart failure may be dominated by acute events, either opportunistic arrhythmias, further episodes of acute myocardial infarction, or repeated exposure to those agents causing the initial myocardial damage (such as alcohol). What is needed is accurate information on the proportion of patients whose disease progresses along those different patterns. To

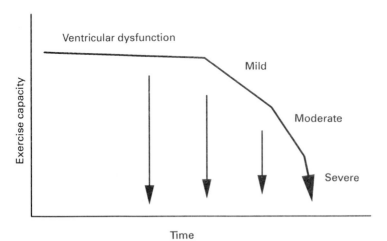

Figure 1.1 The theoretical progression of heart failure. Patients may die either because of gradual worsening of heart failure or because of further events such as an acute myocardial infarction or repeated exposure to the original cause of the heart failure. The proportion of patients with different types of heart failure who follow each course is, as yet, largely unknown.

achieve that end, large long-term studies of entire populations with atheroma are needed. Epidemiological studies of heart failure have, for too long, been the Cinderella of cardiology, an ugly sister being the extensive resources provided for the epidemiological investigation of coronary arterial disease.

2

New nutritional aspects of ischaemic heart disease: polyunsaturated fatty acids and anti-oxidants

Michael F. Oliver

Introduction

The role of individual polyunsaturated fatty acids in the causation of coronary atheroma and of ischaemic heart disease (a term used in this chapter to describe the clinical manifestations of coronary arterial disease) has, until relatively recently, been overshadowed by the well-established positive correlation between the dietary intake of saturated fats and ischaemic heart disease. From the time of the original, and classical, studies of Keys[1], in particular the Seven Countries study, intake of saturated fat and dietary cholesterol have been the focus of most interest. As a result, there have been several national and international reports[2–4] recommending a reduction of dietary saturated fat and of cholesterol.

Most of these have been equivocal about the benefit of increasing the intake of unsaturated fat. One reason has been that the calculated effects on concentrations of cholesterol in the serum produced by reducing dietary saturated fat have been demonstrated to be greater than those of increasing polyunsaturated fats[5,6]. Another is the initial assumption, now recognized as erroneous, that monounsaturated fats play no role in the modulation of atherogenic proteins[7]. Yet another factor has been the obsession of many influential sections of the medical and scientific community with raised blood cholesterol as by far the most important factor in the pathogenesis of ischaemic heart disease.

Fatty acids and coronary atheroma

The reasons why cholesterol accumulates, often extracellularly and in crystalline form, in the arterial wall is a good starting point for this brief review. The experimental evidence is strong that serum concentrations of cholesterol and the low density lipoprotein component of cholesterol are the most powerful determinants of accumulation of cholesterol in the arterial wall. Patients with familial hypercholester-olaemia have a genetic defect of the B/E receptor system for low density lipoprotein which leads to particularly high concentrations of this component in the serum, together with extensive and premature coronary atherosclerosis and premature ischaemic heart disease[8]. Experiments increasing the intake of saturated fat in the diet lead to increases in the low density component of lipoprotein in cholesterol and to coronary atheroma.

Recently, the uptake of low density lipoprotein by receptors in monocytes and macrophages in the arterial endothelium has been shown to be insufficient to lead to extensive formation of foam cells. It has been proposed that the conversion of monocytes or macrophages to foam cells is dependent on the uptake of oxidatively modified low density lipoprotein, and that a modified receptor system also exists[9]. The mechanisms through which oxidative conversion of the lipoprotein occurs, and the sites where it occurs, are now under intensive study.

These new observations should focus our attention on the proportion and nature of the unsaturated fatty acids present in plasma and their esterification to membrane phospholipids in endothelial cells and monocytes and macrophages. In general, the more unsaturated the polyunsaturated fatty acids, the more lipid peroxidation will take place. Interestingly, a powerful anti-oxidant drug, probucol, has a stabilizing effect on oxidized low density lipoprotein uptake[10]. It has also been demonstrated that vitamin E, a naturally-occurring anti-oxidant, has a similar stabilizing effect in cell culture preparations. Therefore, the nature of the polyunsaturated fatty acids present in the arterial wall, in the plasma, and in the diet together with the antioxidant vitamins probably have a much more direct effect on accumulation of cholesterol in the arterial wall than has been thought.

Another area under intensive study is the mechanisms through which the high density lipoprotein 'scavenger' system removes arterial lipid. The experimental and epidemiological evidence is strong that low concentrations of the high density lipoproteins in the plasma favour, while high concentrations appear to protect against, accumulation of cholesterol[11]. It should not be thought, however, that this is an inevitable inverse association, since the mechanisms through which high proportions of low density and low proportions of high density lipoproteins have their specific effects may be different. And so the question arises at the molecular level as to how high density lipoproteins transport cholesterol out of the arterial wall. At the biochemical level, the evidence is impressive for transfer of cholesterol to circulating very low density lipoproteins and to receptors for high density lipoproteins in the liver.

But how is the removal of extracellular cholesterol from the arterial wall implemented? The cholesterol transferase systems, of which there are several, lead to the esterification of cholesterol in preparation for its transport in plasma by high density and very low density lipoproteins, and are, therefore, dependent on the spectrum of fatty acids in the various lipid moieties affected by these systems. The fatty acid composition of circulating lipoproteins and of other plasma cells (such as platelets and monocytes), and also of vascular cells, depends on the relative proportions of phospholipids (with which these fatty acids are esterified) on the surface of and within these cells. The phospholipid composition of lipids in membranes is known to be strikingly different from one type of cell to another and, like fatty acid esterification, will change according to the milieu surrounding the cell and the intracellular functions and requirements of cells.

Fatty acids and ischaemic heart disease

It is unnecessary to review or repeat the evidence[12] indicating the relationship of saturated fatty acids to ischaemic heart disease, but a brief account of some of the newer information concerning the inverse relationship between unsaturated fats and arterial disease might be appropriate. Also, it may be helpful to provide an outline of the metabolic pathways of fatty acids in man (Figure 2.1) and their interrelations (Figure 2.2).

Monounsaturated fatty acids

Previously, monounsaturated fatty acids, particularly oleic acid (C18:1 n-9), were thought to be neutral in respect of atherogenesis and ischaemic heart disease. But now it is clear that oleic acid has a powerful effect in lowering low density lipoproteins and that it, probably, also raises high density lipoproteins[7]. Stearic acid (C18:0) may also have a somewhat similar effect as a result of its rapid metabolism to oleic acid. The beneficial effects of a diet high in olive oil have been suspected for many years and are a potent explanation for the low incidence of ischaemic heart disease in the Mediterranean region.

Polyunsaturated fatty acids

In many countries, such as the USA, Australia and Canada – and more recently the

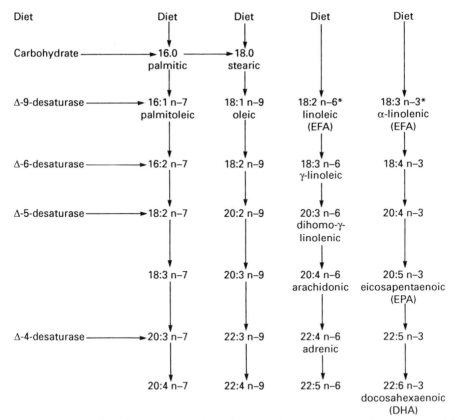

Figure 2.1 An outline of the pathways of metabolism of the n-7, n-9, n-6 and n-3 unsaturated fatty acids and points of action of desaturases. The different series of fatty acids compete with one another, especially at the desaturation steps. At least in part the different series are metabolized by the same enzyme sequences. *Only the n-6 and n-3 fatty acids are essential

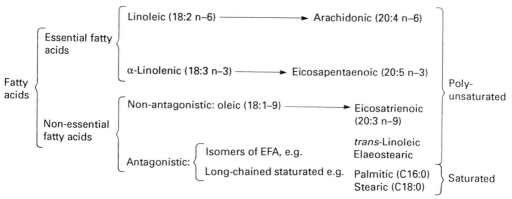

Figure 2.2 The interrelationships between essential fatty acids and other fatty acids (see reference[14])

UK – there has been an impressive reduction in the incidence of ischaemic heart disease. In England and Wales, for example, the reduction during the years 1978–88 and 1987–88 for men under the age of 45 has been in the region of 40%; for men aged 46–55, the decrease has been in the region of 20% and for older men in the region of 10%. Similar figures apply to Scotland. Many views have been advanced to explain these decreases. The main contenders are a change in lifestyle associated with preventive measures and improvement in medical services. Even taking both into account, a proportion of the decrease remains unexplained. Regarding the former – changes in lifestyle – the most striking of all has been a reduction in cigarette smoking. The mechanism through which such reduction may have had a beneficial effect is still not clear.

Another important contributor, regarding lifestyle, is changes in diet. Analysis of international and national dietary returns in relation to changes in incidence of ischaemic heart disease indicate that there has, over the period of reduction of the disease, been only a small and inconsistent decrease in the amount of fat calories consumed and also in the amount of dietary cholesterol taken. The most striking and consistent change has been an increase in these nations in the total consumption of polyunsaturated fats[14].

Omega-6 fatty acids

The vegetable oils – corn, sunflower and safflower oils, for example – are the richest source of linoleic acid, (C18:2 n-6) in the Western diet. Linoleic acid is an essential fatty acid and it contributes 70% of the polyunsaturated fats we usually consume. (For a recent review on essential fatty acids, see reference[14].) The dietary intake of oils rich in linoleic acid is inversely related to social class[15] and is reduced in smokers[16]. These oils lower the concentrations of cholesterol and low density lipoproteins in the serum. A relative dietary deficiency may contribute to higher concentrations of low density lipoproteins and also favour intravascular thrombosis (see below). Linoleic acid is converted to arachidonic acid (C20:4 n-6) by a series of desaturase and chain-lengthening steps (Figure 2.1). One of these (Δ6-desaturase) is partially inhibited by nicotine and alcohol. It is a rate-limiting step, and its activity may be reduced in people prone to coronary arterial disease. This is suggested by the finding that feeding gammalinolenic acid (C18:3 n-6) to men with ischaemic heart disease led to a dose-dependent increase in adipose dihomogammalinolenic acid (C20:3 n-6), whereas the feeding of linoleic acid did not.

Populations with a high incidence of ischaemic heart disease have a low intake of linoleic acid[17]. Also, populations with a relatively low incidence of ischaemic heart disease have a high consumption of linoleic acid and oleic acid. A formal case–control study[18] has assessed the odds ratio of developing angina or myocardial infarction as more than 3:1 in those with the lowest concentrations of linoleate in adipose tissue and platelet membranes. The composition of adipose tissue reflects long-term dietary habits, since the half-life of linoleic acid and adipose tissue is in the region of 10–12 months. There have been three long-term primary prevention trials[19–21] which are consistent in demonstrating that a high polyunsaturated:saturated ratio due to supplementation of the diet with omega-6 fatty acids is associated with a decrease in the incidence of ischaemic heart disease.

Omega-3 fatty acids

Consumption of the other principal family of fatty acids – n-3 fatty acids, contained mostly in fish oils – may also be lower in populations with a high incidence of ischaemic heart disease. The epidemiological evidence is, however, not entirely consistent[22]. Nevertheless, there is a similar inverse relation between eicosapentaenoic acid (C20:5 n-3) with the incidence of angina and myocardial infarction[18] and there is evidence from a prospective controlled trial in patients after myocardial infarction that eating fish twice weekly reduces mortality due to ischaemic heart disease[23]. There is also evidence that n-3 fatty acids can reduce the rate of restenosis after coronary angioplasty and retard the rate of accumulation of atheroma produced experimentally. The mechanisms through which a protective effect of n-3 fatty acids may operate are not clear. The evidence for such an effect has recently been reviewed[24]. They do not decrease either the total or low density lipoprotein component of cholesterol, but may have an effect on myocardial function. Their antithrombotic and antiarrhythmic actions may be the key (see next two sections).

Fatty acids and thrombosis

The experimental evidence is strong that saturated fatty acids favour the development of thrombosis and that polyunsaturated fatty acids protect against it[25,26]. But not all saturated fatty acids have the same effect. Myristic acid (C14:0), for example, exerts a greater adverse effect than stearic acid (18:0). Polyunsaturated fatty acids of the n-6 series are antithrombotic but the exact mechanisms with which they work are unclear[25]. The polyenoic n-3 fatty acids also have an antithrombotic action[26]. They partially displace the n-6 fatty acids – arachidonic acid in particular – from phospholipids of plasma membranes. This substitution results in a decrease of the stimulated production of prostanoids of the 2 series and creates the potential for synthesis of prostanoids of the 3 series. Whether the anti-thrombotic effects of these polyenes is entirely or predominantly related to production of prostanoids is not clear.

A further area of great interest, therefore, is the relationship of raised triglycerides to fibrinogen and factor VIIC – as prothrombotic influences – and to PAI_1 as a determinant of fibrinolysis. In general, the higher the concentration of triglyceride the higher the titres of factor VIIC[27] and the higher the activity of PAI_1[28]. But very little is known about the effect of individual fatty acids, esterified to glyceride-glycerol, and therefore available through increased concentrations of triglyceride as modulators of thrombosis.

Fatty acids and myocardial metabolism

The myocardium is a Cinderella in the field of nutrition and lipids. The fact that it is responsible for ischaemic pain, that it becomes infarcted, and that it develops lethal arrhythmias is often completely overlooked by some epidemiologists and researchers into athenosclerosis!

There is abundant evidence of increased accumulation of triglyceride in the myocardium with advancing age, and of accumulation of triglyceride in areas of ischaemic damage and infarction[29]. Such increased concentrations will form a reserve for release of excess intra-cellular concentrations of free fatty acids when lipolysis is stimulated by catecholamines. In the presence of ischaemia, when lactate and pyruvate are not utilized, such an excess of free fatty acids over the available glucose will stretch even further the requirements of ischaemic tissue for oxygen[30,31].

Not only may there be an adverse overall metabolic effect of accumulation of triglyceride, but myocardial ischaemia and infarction is associated with formation of free radicals[32], particularly during reperfusion[33]. Polyunsaturated fatty acids are specially vulnerable to attack by free radicals: oxidative damage (lipid peroxidation) can result and cause reduction in membrane fluidity and permeability. It is not difficult, therefore, to envisage that an imbalance of fatty acids in the membranes of myocardial cells might have a profound influence on ionic exchange. For example, it is known that ventricular fibrillation induced during ligation of coronary arteries in animals can be prevented by pre-feeding with polyunsaturated fats, particularly n-3 fatty acids[34,35]. The mechanism of protection has yet to be worked out. Ventricular fibrillation in man may be more common when saturated fatty acids are relatively low[36].

Anti-oxidants and fatty acids

Lipid peroxidation caused by attack by free radicals can be terminated and prevented by the action of scavenging molecules of free radicals, such as vitamins E and C[37]. Oxidation of low density lipoproteins occurs more readily with depletion of vitamin E, and also loss of linoleic and arachidonic acids[38]. There is somewhat equivocal epidemiological evidence that populations with a high incidence of ischaemic heart disease have a low intake of vitamin E and C, and vice versa. More convincing is a recent report of a formal case–control study showing a highly significant inverse relation between concentrations of vitamin E and vitamin C in the plasma and the risk of angina pectoris[39]. This is consistent with the finding that between 20% and 25% of middle-aged Scotsmen, in whom the finding of ischaemic heart disease is particularly high, never eat citrus fruit[40]. A low consumption of foods containing vitamin E is associated with a low consumption of linoleic acid (see above), since both are present in cereals.

Dietary implications

The 1984 COMA report[2] was pusillanimous about recommending increases in the consumption of polyunsaturated fats, although the proposal was to increase the ratio with saturated fats to the region of 0.6 within 10 years. Much of this was expected to be achieved by a reduction of saturated fats. Reservations were expressed about the metabolic consequences of the consumption of trans-fatty acids formed during the commercial preparation and partial hydrogenation of vegetable oils. Trans-fatty acids are antagonistic to polyunsaturates and can be metabolized like saturated fats (Figure 2.2).

It now seems clear that the case for increasing the intake of polyunsaturated fat of both the n-6 and n-3 series is stronger. The ideal diet might be one in which 30–35% of total calories comes from fat, with 8–10% from saturated fats, 12–14% from monounsaturated fats and 8–10% from polyunsaturated fats. The common dietary sources of fatty acids are shown in Table 2.1.

The need for supplementation of the diet with anti-oxidants (notably vitamins E and C), particularly in populations with a high incidence of ischaemic heart disease, is indicated partly as a result of the recommendation of an increased intake of polyunsaturated fats and partly because of their probable protective effect on several of the mechanisms described above.

Table 2.1 Common sources of dietary fatty acids

Predominantly saturated	Percentage of TFA	Predominantly n-6	Linoleic* as % of TFA		
Coconut oil	88	Safflower	73		
Cow milk fat	62	Corn oil	57		
Cocoa butter	60	Sunflower seed oil	56		
Human milk fat	50	Cotton seed oil	50		
Beef tallow	48				
Palm oil	48				
		Predominantly n-3	a-linolenic* EPA and DHA as % of TFA		
Egg yolk (also mono)	37	Linseed oil	55		
Lard (also mono)	36	Mackerel oil	27		
Mackerel oil (also n-3)	35	Codliver oil	25		
Chicken fat (also mono)	33	Salmon oil	14		
Predominantly monosaturated		Mixed unsaturated fats	Mono	n-6	n-3
Olive oil	77	New rape seed	64	20	8
Lard	53	Soybean oil	27	51	7
Peanut oil	51	Walnut oil	23	55	11
Chicken fat	49				
Egg yolk	48				
Whale oil (also n-3)	66				
Salmon oil (also n-3)	59				
Codliver oil (also n-3)	54				

* Linoleic (18:2 n-6) and α-linolenic (18:3 n-3) are essential fatty acids.
EPA = eicosapentaenoic or timnodonic acid (20:5 n-3); DHA = docosahexaenoic acid (22:6 n-3); TFA = total fatty acids.

Conclusion

The adverse effects of excess saturated fatty acid are undeniable with regard to both coronary atherosclerosis and ischaemic heart disease. But more attention should be given to the beneficial metabolic actions of polyunsaturated fatty acids. The consequences of any deficiency relative to saturated fats, particularly when availability of anti-oxidants is also reduced, include higher concentrations of low density and lower concentrations of high density lipoproteins; an increased tendency to oxidative modification of low density lipoprotein; a prothrombotic and anti-fibrinolytic action; and a deleterious effect on myocardial metabolism during ischaemia.

An increase in the intake of unsaturated fats (monoenes and polyenes) is indicated and, with this, more of the anti-oxidant vitamins (E and C) should be consumed. This is not a new recommendation for reducing ischaemic heart disease but the evidence for it is increasingly compelling. And it has not been implemented in many countries with continuing high rates of ischaemic heart disease or, with any real consistency, in individuals at high risk.

References

1. Keys, A. Coronary heart disease in seven countries. *Circulation*, **41**, 1–198, 1970
2. Report of the Committee on Medical Aspects of Food Policy. *Diet and Cardiovascular Disease*. DHSS, HMSO, London, 1984
3. European Atherosclerosis Society. Strategies for the prevention of coronary heart disease: a policy statement. *Eur. Heart J.*, **8**, 77–88, 1987
4. National Cholesterol Education Program. Report on detection, evaluation and treatment of high blood cholesterol in adults. *Arch. Intern. Med.*, **148**, 36–69, 1988
5. Hegsted, D.M., McGaudy, R.B., Myers, M.L., *et al.* Quantitative effects of 'dietary fat' on serum cholesterol in man. *Am. J. Clin. Nutr.*, **17**, 281–95, 1965
6. Keys, A., Anderson, J.T. and Grande, F. Serum cholesterol response to changes in the diet 1. Iodine value of dietary fat versus 25-P. *Metabolism*, **14**, 747–758, 1965
7. Grundy, S.M. Comparison of monounsaturated fatty acids and carbohydrates for lowering plasma cholesterol. *N. Engl. J. Med.*, **324**, 745–748, 1986
8. Goldstein, J.L. and Brown, M.S. Familial hypercholesterolaemia. In *Metabolic Basis of Inherited Disease*, 5th edn (eds Stanbury, J.B., Wyngaarden, J.B., Frederickson, D.S., Goldstein, J.L. and Brown, M.S.), McGraw-Hill, New York, pp. 672–712, 1983
9. Steinberg, D., Parthasarathy, S., Carew, T.E., *et al.* Beyond cholesterol – modification of low-density lipoproteins that increase its atherogenicity. *N. Engl. J. Med.*, **520**, 915–923, 1989
10. Parthasarathy, S., Young, S.G., Witztum, J.L., *et al.* Probucol inhibits oxidative modification of low density lipoproteins. *J. Clin. Invest.*, **77**, 641–644, 1986
11. Miller, N.E. High density lipoprotein, atherosclerosis and ischaemic heart disease. *Atherosclerosis: Mechanisms and Approaches to Therapy* (ed. N.E. Miller), Raven Press, New York, pp. 153–168, 1983
12. Haalgren, B. (ed.) *Diet and Prevention of Coronary Heart Disease and Cancer*. Raven Press, New York, 1986
13. Rose, G. Causes of the trends and variations in CHD mortality in different countries. *Int. J. Epidemiol.*, **18**, (Suppl. 1), 174–179, 1989
14. Sinclair, H.M. History of essential fatty acids. In *Omega-6 Essential Fatty Acids* (ed. D.F. Horrabin), Alan R. Liss, New York, pp. 1–21, 1990
15. Fulton, M., Thomson, M., Elton, R.A., Brown, S., Wood, D.A. and Oliver, M.F. Cigarette smoking, social class and nutrient intake: relevance to coronary heart disease. *Eur. J. Clin. Ntur.*, **42**, 797–803, 1988
16. Oliver, M.F. Cigarette smoking, polyunsaturated fats, linoleic acid and coronary heart disease. *Lancet*, **i**, 1241–1243, 1989
17. Riemersma, R.A., Wood, D.A., Butler, S., *et al.* Linoleic acid in adipose tissue and coronary heart disease. *Br. Med. J.*, **292**, 1423–1427, 1986.

18. Wood, D.A., Riemersma, R.A., Butler, S., *et al.* Linoleic and eicosapentaenoic acids in adipose tissue and platelets and risk of coronary heart disease. *Lancet*, **i**, 177–183, 1987
19. Dayton, S., Pearce, M.L., Hashimoto, S., *et al.* A controlled clinical trial of a diet high in unsaturated fat in preventing complications of atherosclerosis. *Circulation*, **XL** (Suppl. II), 1–62, 1969
20. Turpeinen, O., Karvonen, M.J., Pekkarinen, M., *et al.* Dietary prevention of coronary heart disease: The Finnish Mental Hospital Study. Int. J. Epidemiol., **8**, 99–118, 1979
21. Hjermann, I., Holme, I., Velve Byre, K. and Leren, P. Effect of diet and smoking intervention on the incidence of coronary heart disease. Report from the Oslo Study Group of a randomized trial in healthy men. *Lancet*, **ii**, 1303–1310, 1981
22. Sanders, T.A.B. Fish and coronary artery disease. *Br. Heart J.*, **57**, 214–219, 1987
23. Burr, M.L., Fehily, A.M., Gilbert, J.F., *et al.* Effects of changes in fat, fish and fibre intakes on death and myocardial reinfarction: diet; and reinfarction trial. *Lancet*, **ii**, 757–761, 1989
24. Weber, P.C. Atherosclerosis risk factor modification by n-3 fatty acids. *Atherosclerosis Rev.*, **21**, 91–102, 1990
25. Nordoy, A. and Goodnight, S.H. Dietary lipids and thrombosis. *Arteriosclerosis*, **10**, 149–163, 1990
26. Hornstra, G. The significance of fish and fish-oil enriched food for prevention and therapy of ischaemic cardiovascular disease. In *Role of Fats in Human Nutrition*, Academic Press, New York, pp. 152–205, 1989
27. Miller, G.J., Martin, J.C., Webster, J., *et al.* Association between dietary fat intake and plasma Factor VII coagulant activity – a predictor of cardiovascular mortality. *Atherosclerosis*, **60**, 269–277, 1986
28. Wiman, B. and Hamsten, A. The fibrinolytic enzyme system and its role in the etiology of thromboembolic disease. *Sem. Thromb. Haemost.*, **16**, 207–216, 1990
29. Neely, J.R. and Morgan, H.E. Relationship between carbohydrate and lipid metabolism and the energy balance of heart muscle. *Ann Rev. Physiol.*, **36**, 413–490, 1974
30. Kurien, V.A. and Oliver, M.F. A metabolic cause of arrhythmias during acute myocardial hypoxia. *Lancet*, **i**, 813–815, 1970
31. Opie, L.H. Metabolism of free fatty acids, glucose and catecholamines in acute myocardial infarction: Relation to myocardial ischaemia and infarct size. *Am. J. Cardiol.*, **36**, 938–954, 1975
32. McCord, J.M. Oxygen-derived free radicals in post-ischaemic tissue injury. *N. Engl. J. Med.*, **312**, 159–163, 1985
33. Zweier, J.L., Flaherty, J.T. and Weisfeldt, M.L. Direct measurement of free radical generation following reperfusion of ischaemic myocardium. *Proc. Nat. Acad. Sci.*, **84**, 1404–1407, 1987
34. McLennan, P.L., Abeywardena, M.Y. and Charnock, J.S. Influence of dietary lipids on arrhythmias and infarction after coronary artery ligation in rats. *Can. J. Physiol. Pharmacol.*, **63**, 1411–1417, 1985
35. Riemersma, R.A. and Sargent, C.A. Dietary fish oil and ischaemic arrhythmia. *J. Intern. Med.*, **225** (Suppl. 1), 111–116, 1989
36. Abraham, R., Riemersma, R.A., Wood, D.A., *et al.* Adipose fatty acid composition and the risk of serious ventricular arrhythmias in acute myocardial infarction. *Am. J. Cardiol.*, **63**, 269–272, 1989
37. McCay, P.B. Vitamin E: interaction with free radicals and ascorbate. *Ann. Rev. Nutr.*, **5**, 323–340, 1985
38. Esterbauer, H., Jurgens, G., Quehenberger, O. and Kollen, E. Auto-oxidation of human low density lipoprotein: loss of polyunsaturated fatty acids and vitamin E and generation of aldehydes. *J. Lipid Res.*, **28**, 495–509, 1987
39. Riemersma, R.A., Wood, D.A., MacIntyre, C.C.A., *et al.* Risk of angina pectoris and plasma concentration of vitamins A, C and E and carotene. *Lancet*, **i**, 1–5, 1990
40. Tunstall-Pedoe, H., Smith, W.C.S., Crombie, J.K. and Tavendale, R. Coronary risk factor and life style variation across Scotland: results from the Scottish Heart Study. *Scot. Med. J.*, **34**, 556–560, 1989

3

The relevance of magnetic resonance to the management and early diagnosis of coronary vascular disease: the great opportunity for post-Hippocratic medicine

Donald Longmore

Introduction

Medical practice is still based on the principles defined by the School of Hippocrates more than 2400 years ago. We accept the symptomatic sick into our institutions, we do our utmost to make a diagnosis and, when possible, we treat them to the best of our ability. The contents of this volume represent the apogee of contemporary medicine. The various chapters discuss the huge efforts made to manage patients with myocardial damage following coronary occlusion. In most centres, the moral principles defined by Hippocrates are still adhered to, and, within the constraints of contemporary ethics, we behave well towards our patients and teach the next generation our meagre knowledge. Many of us, however, recognize the shortcomings of contemporary medical practice, particularly when applied to the occlusive vascular disease of which half of us are destined to die.

Words from the hippocratic school over 2 millenia old are still pertinent today and worthy of further consideration today:

'Exactness is difficult to achieve and small errors are bound to occur. I warmly commend the physician who makes small mistakes; infallibility is rarely to be seen. Most doctors seem to me to be in the position of poor navigators. In calm weather they can conceal their mistakes, but when overtaken by a mighty storm or a violent gale, it is evident to all that it is their ignorance and error which is the ruin of the ship. So it is with the sorry doctors who are in the great majority. They cure men but slightly ill, in whose treatment even the biggest mistakes would have no serious consequences. Such diseases are many and much more common than the more serious ones. When doctors make mistakes over such cases, their errors are unperceived by the layman, but when they have to treat a serious and dangerous case, a mistake or lack of skill is obvious to all and vengeance for either error is not long delayed.'

From his writings, it appears that Hippocrates recognized the basic shortcoming of medicine and the lack of understanding of the basic problems. In a recent symposium, which formed the kernel for this book, we addressed the all too common problems of how best to manage established occlusive vascular disease which has compromised part of an organ – the heart muscle. Unfortunately, we lack information about the natural history of the disease process, its causative factors, why some are apparently immune, and what lifestyles or drugs might prevent it, or reverse its progress, before the desperate clinical problem arises which is our overall subject. In this book, the diagnosis and management of established coronary arterial disease, and methods of predicting the prognosis of the patient, are discussed in depth. This unhappy position may no longer be inevitable because, with the advent of magnetic resonance, the most powerful diagnostic instrument yet conceived, there is the opportunity to move into the new era of preventing acquired cardiovascular disease. Before magnetic resonance, there was little chance of understanding the natural history of common disease processes, notably the development of atheroma. There was no practical method of monitoring the efficacy of preventive or therapeutic methods. Clinical trials depend on a clear, definable end point, such as reinfarction or death. Therefore, large numbers of patients need to be studied over a long period of time at great cost. What little understanding we have of the natural history of occlusive vascular disease is based on risk factors. Attempts to correlate risk factors with the incidence of cardiovascular disease are the norm. The correlations, however, are always limited and the proponents of the philosophy of risk factors must admit that they may not even be aware of the major factors. Careful correlation of normal ranges of cardiovascular structure and function in the normal and in those with presently undetectable presymptomatic disease, established by magnetic resonance, will offer much more powerful studies of the factors influencing disease.

Everybody knows that occlusive vascular disease and lung cancer correlate with smoking. How many, however, remember that lung cancer also correlates significantly with coffee drinking, with intake of sugar, eating of spicy food, a high rate of sexual intercourse, with bodily habits, with personality, and with emotional type? These correlations suggest that there must be many other factors as yet unknown, notably the genetic make-up which is at the heart of the correlation. The genes are the predisposing factors. Some of the other correlations are multipliers − including smoking, one of the most powerful multipliers of all. As doctors in our present state of ignorance, we are justified in a blanket condemnation of smoking. We are right to advise every patient to give it up but, as biologists, we must be fascinated by the fact that some are more susceptible than others, with the knowledge that occasional people chain-smoke all their lives and live a full life without developing cancer, bronchitis, emphysema, occlusive vascular disease, bladder cancer or any of the other ailments that correlate with smoking. In the same way, there appear to be people who can gorge on cholesterol-rich foods, grow obese and never suffer a hint of vascular occlusion. On the other hand, there are slim, fit patients who do all the right things yet fall victim to coronary occlusion. The classical response to this seeming injustice, the effects of fate, is now no longer acceptable. The onset of vascular occlusion is not stochastic but the result of multiple aetiological factors in our make-up, environment and behaviour. If we can use magnetic resonance to study the normal, and to pin down these factors for each disease, we could use it to turn medicine into a truly predictive science. No longer will we need to tell a patient that he has a number of risk factors which may cause his vital arteries to block. Instead, we may be able to tell each individual, for example, that he must change his lifestyle or he will inevitably succumb; or, on the other hand, that his chances of major cardiovascular disease, if he continues in the same way, are so remote that he can disregard them.

Calm weather

In its traditionally reactionary way, the medical profession has already uncomfortably weathered waters ruffled by many advances that have come from without the profession, all of which have changed medical practice superficially without changing the principles. These advances include anaesthetics and antibiotics from chemists, transplantation from biologists, X-rays from physicists, steroids from biochemists, the contraceptive pill from pharmacologists, extracorporeal circulation from engineers, pacemakers from electronic engineers, implants from metallurgists and plastics technologists and, now, magnetic resonance from nuclear physicists and chemists.

The storm and the great gales yet to come

Better education and higher standards of living but, most importantly, the quantum leap in technology for communication in the Western world following World War II have raised public expectation from medicine. Survival is no longer the prime consideration. There are public and political pressures for a better quality of life. The demographic shift towards a large 'active retired' population has increased demand for life-enhancing, as well as life-saving, medicine. The ever more enlightened public are beginning to ask questions about management of disease. Is medical technology, which receives so much publicity in the twilight years of the twentieth century, being properly managed?

Failed prevention

Nowhere is the philosophy of managing established symptomatic illness with high technology, advanced surgery and sophisticated pharmacological agents better illustrated than in the management of acquired cardiovascular disease. The medical management varies dramatically when a blockage occurs in an artery of a vital organ. If the artery happens to affect the brain and causes stroke, management of the patient is little different from what it might have been at the time of Galen. But, when the history is suggestive of coronary arterial disease, the full panoply of high-technology medical management, some of which is described in this volume, is unleashed. The management of patients with symptomatic heart disease depends on clinical diagnosis followed by invasive diagnosis. In so far as it goes, the diagnostic method is adequate. A patient who has been through the routine is likely to have a comprehensive anatomical diagnosis but there are still major gaps in the information about the physiology of the compromised heart muscle. Coronary angiography, the cornerstone of assessment of coronary function, is known, even by its proponents, to be dependent on the skill of those interpreting the images. Here there is a great deal of interobserver variability. A review of contemporary treatment reveals less certainty. Angioplasty is still not always a permanent cure. Coronary arterial surgery, in its various forms, carries a small but significant mortality rate and risk of brain damage[1]. There is still debate about the long-term effects of coronary arterial vein grafts on mortality and concern about the side-effects. Despite these reservations, open-heart surgery for occlusive coronary arterial disease, with about 130 000 operations annually in the USA, has a clear lead over hysterectomy and appendicectomy, hitherto the most popular operations. Possibly this unquestioned pursuance of a potentially flawed series of procedures relates to a huge medical industry supplying cardiodiagnostic equipment, bypass apparatus and monitoring equipment for open-heart surgery and intensive care which creates an additional force resisting the change of focus from the treatment to the prevention of occlusive vascular disease.

The enlightened public are now asking why they pay more and more for the medical care of catastrophe and why they are not benefiting from medical check-ups.

Why is there no satisfactory screening of the population to warn them about impending disease? Fundamental questions are being asked by Governments of less affluent countries about the efficacy of Western medical practice. Should they invest an ever-increasing proportion of their small gross domestic product to copy Western high-technology 'curative' medicine? Is it cost-effective? Has it been shown to work? Every medical student is taught on the basis that curative procedures are effective. All doctors leave medical school knowing that tuberculosis was conquered by mass X-ray and antibiotics. An examination of the incidence of tuberculosis, which has been well documented in England and Wales from 1853 to the present day, shows no deviations from the straight-line decline of the disease apart from the periods of two world wars (Figure 3.1). There are no demonstrable effects of the Public Health Acts, the use of sanatoria, artificial pneumothorax, thoracoplasty, phrenic crush, lobectomy, mass X-ray, streptomycin, isoniacid, PAS. Certainly diseases characterized by both a deep understanding of their natural history and availability of a therapeutic agent have been relegated to the history books, like smallpox and poliomyelitis.

High increasing spending on the management of coronary arterial disease, in contrast, does not appear to be effective. There is no discernible relationship between the incidence and survival from coronary arterial disease and the proportion of national wealth spent on curative medicine. The USA, spending the largest proportion of its gross domestic product, and the UK, nearly the lowest proportion, have a very high incidence of deaths due to coronary arterial disease; whereas France, a high spender, and Japan, the lowest spender in the developed world, share a low incidence. Life expectancy in Japan has increased rapidly from 1965 to 1986. It rose by 7.5 years for men and 8 years for women.

Unless the medical profession takes every opportunity to prevent the major killing

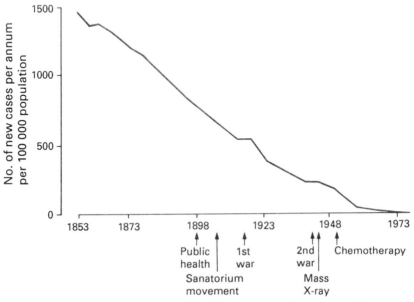

Figure 3.1 The incidence of tuberculosis has fallen steadily in England and Wales since 1853. The only two deviations from the straight line relate to World War I and World War II. There are no discernible effects from medical intervention

diseases, it is at the risk of being overtaken by the mighty storm of protest forecast by Hippocrates, not as a result of mistakes, lack of skills or the general will to try harder, but about the way it conducts its affairs now there appears to be a viable alternative.

Magnetic resonance – the new instrument for accurate navigation

The problem that hitherto faced those in medicine who wish to change the philosophy of medical practice from the management of death to the provision of a lifetime without the blight of accelerated degeneration of the vascular system has been the lack of a reliable method of obtaining essential information about the presymptomatic and very early stages of the disease process. Large numbers of people undergo routine medical examinations, many of which are well conducted using 'state of the art' technology. They can, however, only detect existing end-stage disease and do not appear to be predictive. All know the story that highlights the problems of conventional cardiology applied to coronary arterial disease. The nurse in the preventive clinic rushes in to say, 'Doctor, doctor, the patient you just said was fit has dropped dead on the steps'. The doctor replies, 'Quick, turn him round so that it looks as if he is coming in!'

If magnetic resonance, and new powerful non-invasive techniques, are to achieve their promise as comprehensive cardiovascular diagnostic instruments and tools to screen a population, original thinking and not re-hashed applications of present-day measurements and concepts will be needed. There is little incentive from within medicine to develop and teach ideas that will enable change. Advance may be forced on the profession by demand from an enlightened public with no vested interests other than its own well-being. Rather than deciding whether magnetic resonance can be used to mimic existing tests and whether X-ray based procedures can be replaced by quantitative magnetic resonance studies*, the following questions should be addressed. Is occlusive vascular disease an inescapable part of the ageing process or is it preventable? What is the natural history of the atherogenic process before it produces symptoms? Are preventive and therapeutic measures likely to arrest, or even reverse, the formation of lethal plaques? Can the use of magnetic resonance answer these questions? Undoubtedly, these fundamental questions will not be answered affirmatively unless the medical profession uses new diagnostic capability wisely. Magnetic resonance should not be regarded as just another competitor for computed tomography used for examining less than 7% of all disease. It should not be regarded as an alternative to nuclear medicine, positron emission tomography or diagnostic ultrasound. Its potential may be far greater. As well as doctors using newly-found diagnostic powers intelligently, there is a vital need for the manufacturers to rethink the design of the machines, changing them from being optimized as head scanning machines into those optimized for cardiovascular diagnosis. There would be little point in using magnetic resonance in an attempt to understand occlusive vascular disease if there were not strong indications that this is not just an inescapable part of the ageing process. We do not need reminding that nearly half of

---

*Already some interventions are done using ultrasound. When open-access, real-time, three-dimensional magnetic resonance is available, there will be no case for exposing patients (and medical staff) to ionizing radiation.

the readers of this volume in the UK and the USA will die prematurely of blocked arteries.

Yet, perhaps a reminder is needed that premature death and diminution of the quality of life should be avoidable. Clues about the causative factors in occlusive vascular disease can be found in recent history. The incidence of coronary arterial disease varies from place to place in people of similar race. It also varies from time to time in the same place, indicating that external factors influence its occurrence. After the First World War, the population of Central Europe was poorly nourished and the recorded incidence of occlusive vascular disease was extremely rare. Post-mortem studies in the London Hospital (Whitechapel) starting just after the turn of the century showed a gradual rise in the incidence of coronary arterial disease until the Second World War, when the incidence of coronary arterial disease in the UK fell sharply, only to rise again after the war. After the siege of Leningrad, it was noted that there was little occlusive vascular disease in the survivors. The populations of the concentration camps who survived to be liberated at the end of the Second World War were studied, and post mortems on those who subsequently died showed a remarkably low incidence of occlusive vascular disease. (These groups were starving and highly stressed, calling into question the accepted wisdom about stress.) People with wasting diseases do not have occlusive vascular disease.

In the Korean War, post mortems on soldiers killed in combat revealed a high incidence of coronary arterial disease which, at that time, were thought to be remarkable in such a young age group. Similar findings occurred when American casualties in Vietnam were studied. Severe arterial disease, including ischaemic heart disease, is not unknown in young people and may occur in children, particularly in families with abnormally high levels of blood cholesterol. It appears, therefore, that our genetic make-up and diet contribute to cardiovascular disease.

Many theories are propounded about the causative factors of this process of disease, but it has proved to be too complex to be understood by weak, contemporary techniques, like the study of risk factors. Before considering the methods that might be applied using magnetic resonance for its early detection and gaining an understanding of its natural history, it is important to examine the pathological processes that might be detected with the techniques used for magnetic resonance, and to review the capabilities and limitations of the technique.

Relevant pathology

The discovery in 1976 of prostacyclin by Sir John Vane allowed a new insight into the formation of atheroma, which is highly relevant to magnetic resonance angiography, flow, compliance, pulse wave velocity and chemical shift techniques. (The first human magnetic resonance image was also produced in 1976 by Professor Peter Mansfield in Nottingham.)

One aspect of atherogenesis may be related to an aberration of the normal clotting mechanism on which we depend for survival. When a blood vessel is cut, the traumatized area does not produce prostacyclin, endothelial derived relaxation factor (EDRF) or, possibly, other protective substances. This allows platelets that stream into the breach to adhere to the sides of the cut and rapidly form a plaque to staunch the flow of blood. The platelets quickly break down and secrete platelet derived growth factor (PDGF). This hormone has the remarkable property of causing smooth muscle in the blood vessel wall to grow rapidly to repair the cut. If, for some reason (as yet unknown), an area of the wall of the blood vessel fails to secrete prostacyclin, platelets from the blood adhere to it as if it were a cut. The adherent disintegrating platelets secrete their growth factor which stimulates the smooth muscle, causing it to grow as if it were healing a cut. The smooth muscle grows into the only available space, the lumen of the vessel, and partially blocks the vessel. Following this event, the smooth muscle usually regresses and the incident passes unnoticed. Occasionally, however, as is demonstrated by indium-labelled platelets, the plaque remains as an active site for adherence of platelets, and the stimulation of smooth muscle continues. Sometimes, the plaques become the site of deposition of lipid, and an atheromatous plaque can contain up to 28% lipid.

Before examining the potential of magnetic resonance with relation to measuring velocity and changes in acceleration across an atheromatous plaque as a method of detecting it, visualization of the plaques, and chemical analysis of them to obtain the content of lipid, it is necessary` to have an understanding of the capabilities of magnetic resonance. The Appendix to this chapter provides a simplified description of the mechanics of magnetic resonance, which may be studied if the reader wishes to know more about the techniques that are alluded to. A more comprehensive description of the principles of magnetic resonance can be found in the *British Medical Bulletin*[2].

Anatomical studies

Images from magnetic resonance are usually obtained from multiple acquisitions. Each acquisition contributes data to the whole of the picture which is not built up line by line like a TV image. The greater the number of acquisitions, the better the ratio of signal to noise. (The radio signal used to contribute to a voxel in the image comes from the relevant volume in the body, whereas the radio noise comes from the whole patient and the receiver system.) Each acquisition triggers at a constant delay from the R wave, taking up to 4 minutes to provide each set of images. Up to 64 slices can be obtained in each heartbeat. Unfortunately, images built up over many heartbeats are often degraded because sinus arrhythmia, changes in the cybernetic system, and other factors, cause misregistration. These shortcomings are overcome by the use of rapid imaging techniques described below. The images are thin (2–3 mm) tomographic slices in any chosen plane with pixel sizes in cardiac studies down to 0.3×0.3 mm. In still organs, a resolution of $150 \times 150 \times 1000\,\mu m$ is already achievable. Conventional, transverse, sagittal and coronal sections are not suitable for the heart, which lies obliquely in the chest. Similarly, they are not appropriate for studying most vessels which need to be seen in longitudinal or transverse section. It is, therefore, necessary to use a diagnostic strategy optimized to study the heart. A transverse siting image at the level of the middle of the left ventricle is used to measure its angle to the left (Figure 3.2a). From this, a single oblique image is produced in the vertical long axis (Figure 3.2b). This is then used to measure the angle downwards of the left ventricle. From these two angles, a double-oblique plane can be selected which produces a horizontal long axis view of the heart (Figure 3.2c), sometimes termed a 'five-chambered' view. This plane shows the right atrium, the tricuspid valve, the right ventricle, the left atrium, the mitral valve, the left ventricle and its outflow tract. In a good image, the right and left coronary arteries and the coronary sinus may also be seen in the atrioventricular grooves. (They are also well seen in conventional transverse images as they arise from the root of the aorta and

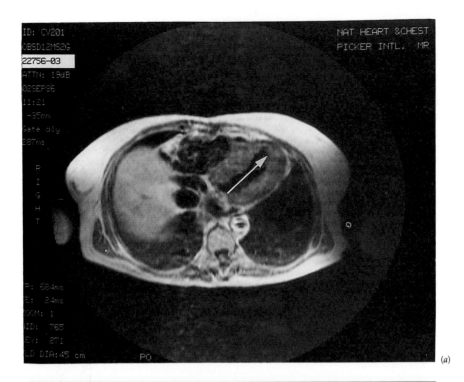

(a)

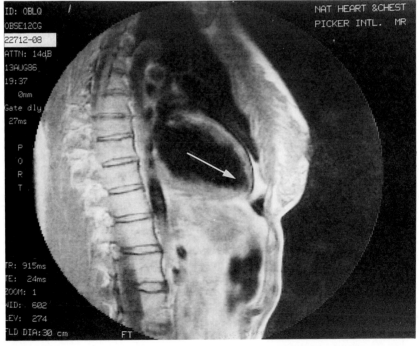

(b)

Figure 3.2 (*a*) A transverse sighting shot across the middle of the left ventricle. The line shows the angle to the left which is used to produce a single oblique image in the vertical long axis. (*b*) A vertical long axis image along the left ventricle. From this, the angle downwards of the left ventricle can be measured, as shown by the arrow, to produce a horizontal long axis double oblique image, shown in (*c*). (*c*) A horizontal long axis 'five-chambered' view of the heart, with a right atrium (RA), the tricuspid valve (TV), the right ventricle (RV), the right coronary artery (RCA), the descending

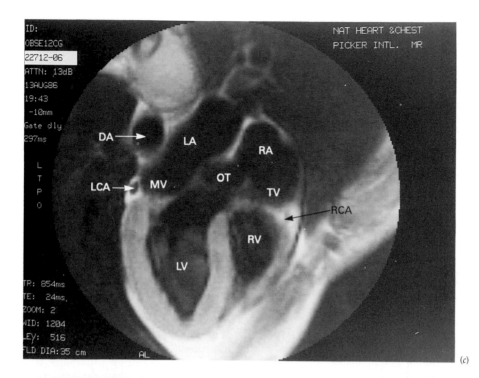

(c)

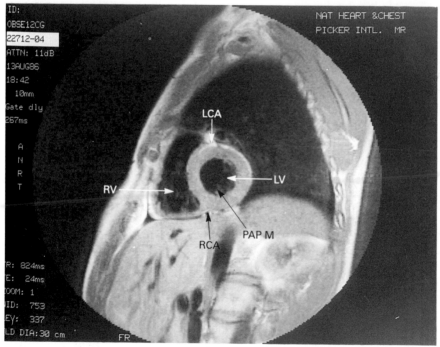

(d)

aorta (DA), the left atrium (LA), the mitral valve (MV), the left ventricle (LV) and the outflow tract (OT). The left coronary artery (LCA) is also indicated. If further detail is required or left ventricular studies are to be undertaken, a further double-oblique image is produced in the short axis. (*d*) A short-axis, double-oblique image of the heart, half-way down the ventricles, showing the left ventricle with the beginnings of the papillary muscles with the right ventricle applied to the front of it. The left and right coronary arteries can be seen end-on. PAPM = papillary muscle

run into the atrioventricular grooves.) If further detail of the ventricular mass is required, images taken in planes perpendicular to the horizontal long axis produce short axis images looking up the barrels of the two ventricles (Figure 3.2d).

Anatomical information can be obtained using two rapid imaging techniques to produce images very much more quickly. One, known as FLASH (fast low-angle shot imaging), uses small flip angles, allowing the T1 relaxation to return to zero in a short period of time and rapid repetition of the sequence. Thus, in 100 ms or so, a reasonable image can be produced. The second, known as EP or echo planar, is a much more sophisticated technique which relies on rapid switching of the gradients using a similar image reconstruction to conventional imaging. This means that 64 sets of information can be obtained in as many milliseconds. Using both techniques, velocity can be encoded, though the results are far more accurate from echo planar imaging and, ultimately, better images can be produced. Rapidly acquired images are not yet of such high quality as conventional images but, because they overcome the degradation described above, they may contain more information. As an alternative, data from magnetic resonance can be acquired in the form of a three-dimensional block. Pathology following coronary arterial occlusion can be seen on the anatomical images, and some problems associated with transplantation can be diagnosed without further investigation. One advantage of diagnosis using magnetic resonance is that, because it is totally non-invasive and not unpleasant for the patient, the tests can be repeated frequently and trends can be observed.

Although an anatomical diagnosis can sometimes be made from a still image, it is usually better to use moving images which can be produced at intervals as short as 10 ms. Movement confers a number of advantages. The eye integrates a signal from anatomical structures in a moving image whilst instinctively rejecting noise. However good a still image may be, it may miss a critical part of the cardiac cycle when a structural abnormality, such as an obstruction in an outflow tract, may be significant. Flow through the coronary arteries is phasic, and a still image taken at a point in the cardiac cycle may miss a coronary artery. The most important advantage of moving images is that they contain information about function of the myocardium, valves and coronary vessels.

Functional information

By the time coronary insufficiency has produced demonstrable anatomical changes, severe muscle damage or muscle death must have occurred. (Figure 3.3(a) and (b) shows a left ventricle which appears to be nearly normal in diastole but is aneurysmal in systole.) Functional assessment of the ventricular muscle, however, both with and without pharmacological stress, can yield more information about that muscle which is still alive but which has a compromised blood supply.

Some information about cardiac function in all the cardiac chambers can be obtained from pairs of still images acquired at end systole and end diastole. From these, ventricular stroke volume and the ejection fraction can be calculated. Wall motion can be studied, giving information both about global cardiac function and areas where the wall is akinetic or dyskinetic. The function of the atriums can be measured from images taken during diastole before atrial contraction starts and after atrial contraction but before ventricular contraction. (Most cardiodiagnosis is based on measurement of left ventricular function. Right ventricular function is less available for study and the atriums are virtually inaccessible.)

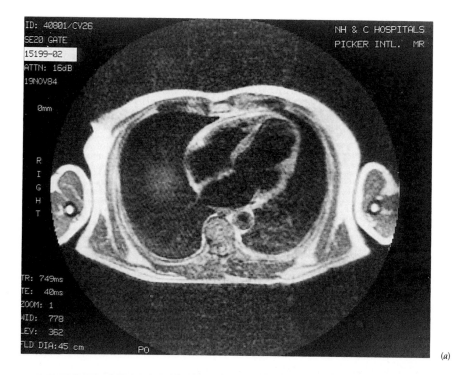

(a)

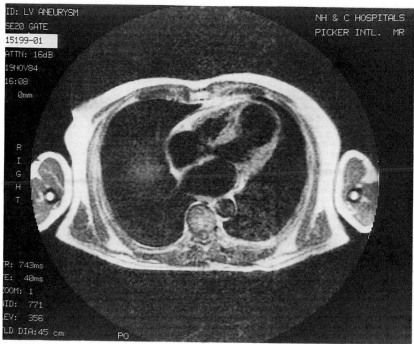

(b)

Figure 3.3 (a) A transverse image of the heart in diastole showing some thinning of the apex of the left ventricle. (b) The corresponding systolic image showing normal thickening of the upper part of the left ventricle and paradoxical movement with aneurysmal dilatation of the apex of the left ventricle

Moving images yield similar information about global ventricular function to that obtained from systolic and diastolic still images, but have the advantages that regional wall motion can be studied and atrial function can be seen. More information about function can be obtained when the heart is stressed. (It is difficult to exercise a patient in the confines of the magnet.) Pharmacological stress can be used either with the administration of dipyridamole (Persantin) or dobutamine[3]. These drugs have the effect of increasing cardiac activity and dilating sound coronary arteries, possibly stealing, by reduction in perfusion, pressure flow from compromised vessels. A heart that appears to be contracting normally in the unstressed state can often be seen to be grossly abnormal when stressed. Areas of ventricular myocardium, which appear to be contracting normally, become akinetic or may even move paradoxically. These changes are best seen in the short axis views and are illustrated in Figure 3.4(a–d) which shows systole and diastole before and after dipyridamole injection.

Magnetic resonance angiography (without velocity encoding)

The techniques using magnetic resonance described above all use signal from the myocardium, vessel walls and still tissues. Moving blood in vessels and the cavities of the heart normally gives no signal, producing 'flow voids' on the image (though

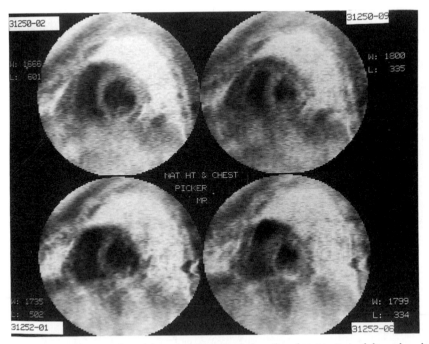

Figure 3.4 (a) A short axis diastolic view of the heart before the administration of dipyridamole. (b) The corresponding systolic image showing apparently normal ventricular contraction. (c) The same heart in diastole after the administration of dipyridamole showing no abnormality. (d) A systolic image of the same heart after the administration of dipyridamole showing an abnormal area of contraction on the upper surface of the left ventricle.

slow-moving blood in cardiac chambers can give a signal mimicking the myocardium). There is often slow moving or static blood overlying an infarcted segment of myocardium. The field even echo re-phasing sequence[4] can be used, as can some other sequences, to produce high signal from moving blood. Blood images in a series of contiguous tomographic slices can be stacked to produce three-dimensional images simulating angiograms. Techniques can then be used to rotate them to give some insight into the vascular tree, the cardiac cavities and the major pulmonary vessels. Figure 3.5 shows an image of a right coronary artery obtained with this technique.

Unfortunately, magnetic resonance angiographic images share, together with conventional X-ray angiography, digital subtraction, and so on, all the problems associated with interpretation. Assessment is subjective and inter-observer variability is a well-known and documented hazard. Vessels that are completely absent may be missed, and the assessment of the significance of a stenosis is open to error. These problems can be partially overcome by encoding velocity, acceleration and higher orders like 'jerk' into image obtained from blood.

Magnetic resonance angiography (with velocity encoding)

Magnetic resonance imaging has a unique advantage. The signal that is used to produce an image is based on a natural radio signal emanating from the protons

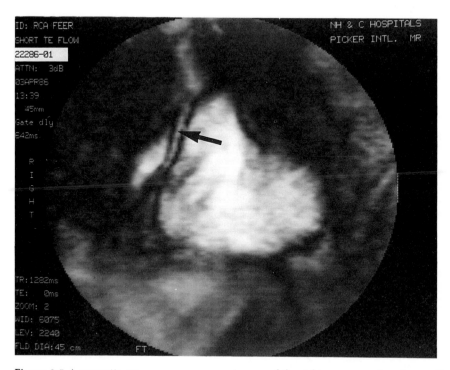

Figure 3.5 A magnetic resonance coronary angiogram of the right coronary artery (arrowed) coming from the right sinus of Valsalva and passing down between the right atrial appendage and the right ventricular outflow tract. One branch to the right ventricle can be seen

which are precessing in unison in the magnetic field. The radio signal has three variables:

1. Frequency, which is used to obtain spatial resolution (the rate of precession relates to the magnetic field strength and during the production of an image each point in the volume of interest has a unique field strength and therefore a unique frequency.
2. Amplitude, which relates to the number of protons in the voxel which is being analysed.
3. Phase, which is the relationship of the signal to its position on the radio wave.

Velocity can be encoded in the phase of the signal. Phase-mapping depends on an application of a magnetic gradient in the direction of expected flow (or at a known angle to it) which will change the phase of still, slow-moving, or fast-moving material. The gradient is applied for a finite time, and is then reversed for the same period of time. Still material is re-phased, but slow-moving material will have moved into a new phase territory, and fast-moving material will have moved further. The problem with simple phase-mapping of this type relates to the fact that the machine is unable to distinguish between the movement of the signal along a sine-wave and its transference to a subsequent wave. In order to overcome this, the field even echo re-phasing technique was developed. This sequence compresses the phase change at the second echo so that it is all contained within one wave (see 'spin echo' in the Appendix). Recently, the technique has been developed to obtain signal at the second echo in times of as short as 3.6 m/s[5]. Figure 3.6 shows a series of velocities

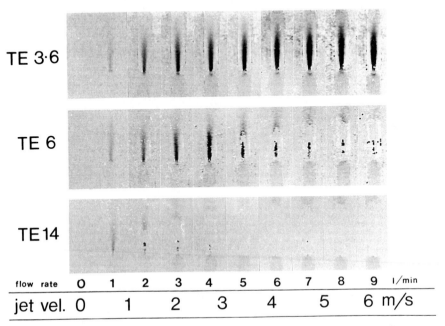

Figure 3.6 Flows up to 6 m/s through a stenosis in a phantom. Signal drop-out at long TE times is clearly seen and good signal from which velocity analysis can be made is obtained at TE 3.6

up to 6 m/s through a stenosis in a phantom at different echo times, showing the importance of very short echo times for the accurate measurement of high velocities. This advance means that velocities up to 6 m/s can be measured to an accuracy of better than 5%. It may be possible to develop techniques using velocity mapping to measure very low flows to assess perfusion of tissues. The measurement of velocity has been validated by a four-way comparison between the stroke volume of the right and left ventricles, and measurement of flow in the pulmonary trunk and aorta (the aortic flow is lower because of the take-off of the coronary arteries)[6,7].

Accurate measurement of velocity can be combined with accurate measurement of the diameter of a stenosis or valve to measure a gradient. Figure 3.7 shows a stenosed mitral valve seen end-on and the velocity profile across it at peak flow. From this, a gradient of 15 mm Hg was measured.

Velocity measurement across or along a vessel can given an insight into its function. Figure 3.8(a) shows the site of anastomosis in a transplanted lung. Figure 3.8(b) shows a velocity profile through the anastomosis of the right pulmonary artery of a transplanted lung to the native artery. Figure 3.8(c) shows the total flow through the pulmonary trunk, the flow through the transplanted right lung and the flow through the native lung. The transplanted lung is taking most of the flow and blood is passing across the pulmonary artery from the native to the transplanted lung during diastole.

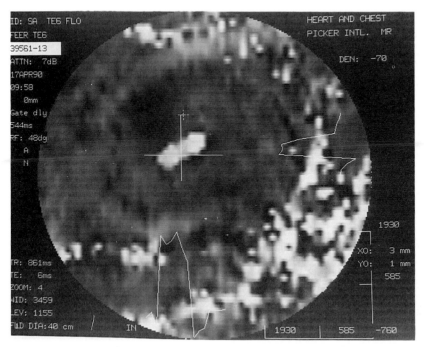

Figure 3.7 A mitral valve seen end-on. Velocity profiles have been measured showing peak flow from which a gradient of 15 mm Hg was calculated

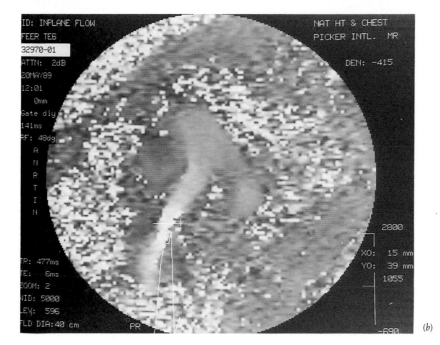

Figure 3.8

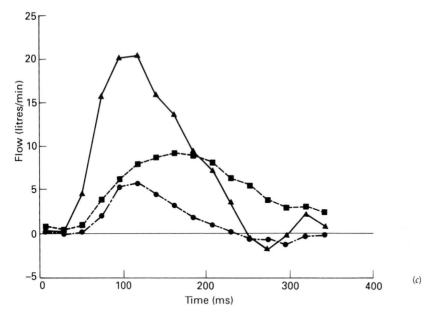

Figure 3.8 (*a*) The site of the anastomosis to a transplanted lung is arrowed. (*b*) A velocity profile through the anastomosis of the right pulmonary artery of a transplanted lung to the native pulmonary artery showing an increase in velocity which indicates a gradient of approximately 20 mm Hg. (*c*) A composite graph of flow curves showing total flow in the pulmonary trunk, flow through the native lung and through the transplanted lung. During diastole, the transplanted lung is taking flow from the native lung. ▲———▲ = pulmonary trunk; ■–––■ = right pulmonary artery; ●–––● = left pulmonary artery.

Tissue characterization (proton imaging)

All conventional magnetic resonance images are maps of proton density (water), although the emphasis can be changed to highlight T1 and T2 relaxation times (see references in Appendix). Tissue oedema can be detected by a change in measured T1 or T2. Both usually increase following a myocardial infarction. Tissue characterization has been studied widely to assess the extent of an infarct, and to determine the extent of stunned myocardium. Unfortunately, the results vary from machine to machine. Although this is a sensitive method of detecting an increase in water in the tissues, oedema is not a very early feature of infarction and the published results are disappointing.

Tissue characterization (sodium imaging)

Although sodium imaging is at an experimental stage, an increase in sodium within the tissues apparently anticipates frank oedema. Most machines used for magnetic resonance can be modified to make them capable of imaging sodium, promising a more sensitive technique for the detection and monitoring of infarction.

Atheroma and chemical shift

Myocardial infarction is a result of the atheromatous process in the coronary vessels. The significance of magnetic resonance for its prevention and management depends on the answer to three questions.

1. Can magnetic resonance detect generalized atheroma?
2. Can magnetic resonance visualize atheromatous plaques?
3. If plaques are seen, is it possible to determine whether they are fibrous end-stage lesions or whether they are active lesions rich in lipid?

Fortunately, the answer to all these questions is yes.

Vascular compliance

Normally, the heart ejects into a complaint (elastic) arterial system whether it is systemic or pulmonary. Generalized atheromatous disease decreases the compliance. This compromises the heart in two ways. First, it has to eject into an inelastic system at a higher pulse wave velocity, therefore increasing its work. Second, an inelastic aortic arch contributes less to the backflow in the aortic root for coronary perfusion[8,9]. Magnetic resonance can be used to measure compliance in the aorta in two ways. First, by measuring directly the difference in the volume of the aorta between peak systole and end diastole related to the pulse pressure, as shown in Figure 3.9. Second, by measuring indirectly the time taken for the pulse wave to travel from the root of the aorta to the descending aorta. The velocity of the pulse wave is the reciprocal of the compliance. Athletes and the very fit retain a high compliance throughout life. In the normal, compliance decreases with age and, in those with arteriopathy, the compliance is prematurely reduced[10] (Figure 3.10). The elasticity of the pulmonary arteries can be observed, but the compliance cannot be calculated because the pulse pressure cannot be measured non-invasively[11]. The fate of a heart after infarction depends in part on the after-load to which it is subjected. Since it is known that the atheromatous process is arrestable and reversible with suitable dietary and therapeutic measures, it is important to determine whether the patient has active plaques and to monitor the efficacy of measures to contain the atheromatous process.

Visualization and analysis of atheromatous plaques

High-resolution spin echo imaging can be used to show plaques[12,13]. Figure 3.11(a) shows an atheromatous plaque at the bifurcation of the aorta. Figure 3.11(b) is the corresponding conventional angiogram. Figure 3.11(c) shows the haemodynamic significance of the plaque. The images from magnetic resonance contain more information than do the angiographic images because they show the plaque, the vessel wall and the surrounding tissues instead of just the lumen. The velocity profile in the aorta shows velocities within the normal range. Velocity is increased on the right side, where the narrowing is less, and greater on the left where the narrowing is clinically significant. A limitation of angiography is the dependence of the significance of a stenosis on interpretation of the significance of a stenosis by a clinician. Mapping of velocity produces accurate numerical data about flow throughout the

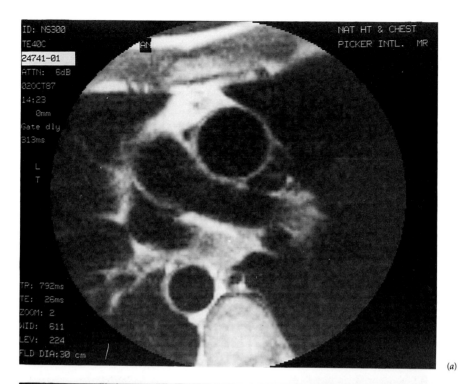

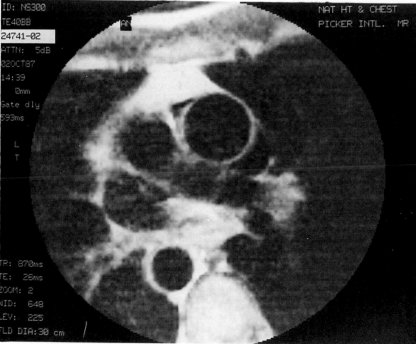

Figure 3.9 (*a*) A systolic image of the ascending and descending aorta. The ascending aorta has a cross-sectional area of 7.1 cm² in systole. (*b*) A diastolic image corresponding to (*a*). The cross-sectional area of the descending aorta is 6.1 cm².

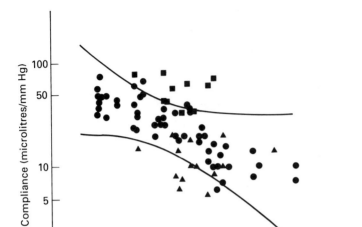

Figure 3.10 The reduction in compliance in the ascending aorta with age showing how athletes retain a good compliance and patients with coronary artery disease (CAD) have a reduced compliance. ● = normals; ■ = athletes; ▲ = patients with CAD.

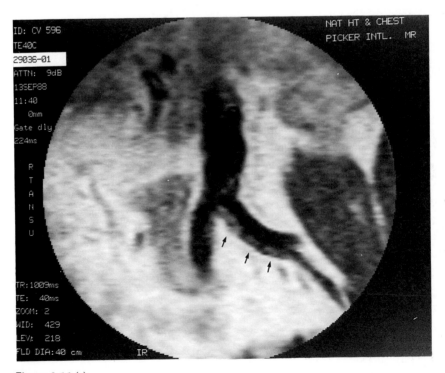

Figure 3.11 (*a*)

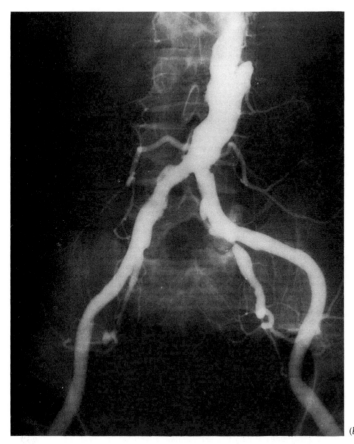

(b)

Figure 3.11 (a) An atheromatous plaque at the bifurcation of the aorta with secondary plaques (arrowed). The corresponding conventional angiogram is shown in (b). (b) A conventional angiogram of the region shown in the magnetic resonance image in (a). There is less information in the X-ray image, which shows only the lumen of the vessel, whereas the magnetic resonance image shows the wall as well. (c) The haemodynamic significance of the plaque illustrated in (a) and (b). There is a normal velocity profile in the descending aorta. The velocity in the right common iliac artery, which would be expected to be slightly lower than the velocity in the aorta, is in fact increased. The velocity in the left common iliac artery (the side on which the patient has symptoms) is further increased, indicating a tight stenosis well seen on the MR image and less well seen on the angiogram

cardiac cycle which can be used in several ways. The total volume of flow to the perfused organ can be measured for each heartbeat or for a given unit of time. This, however, may not be an entirely reliable method of assessing perfusion, because changes in the circulation, notably in the pulsitility and heart rate, can change the nature of flow past an obstruction from laminar to turbulent, thereby increasing loss of energy and reducing perfusion of the tissues.

Velocity mapping can be used to detect a stenosis, either by searching the length of a vessel for increase in velocity which takes place at the site of a narrowing or by measuring acceleration upstream of the obstruction and deceleration downstream. The velocity of blood in paired vessels, such as the carotids arteries, the right and left

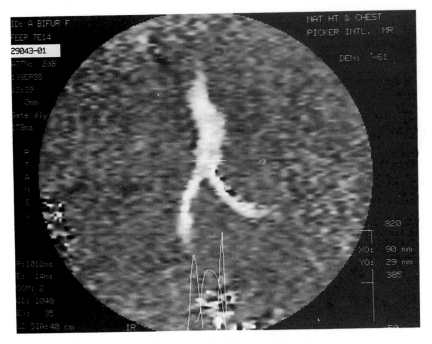

Figure 3.11 (*c*)

coronary arteries, the iliac and renal vessels, and so on, is normally identical on both sides. Any increase in velocity on one side indicates the presence of a stenosis. Figure 3.12(a–c) illustrates this physiological point. It shows cross-sections of the pelvis in a patient with thromboangitis obliterans migrans (Berger's disease). The patient had the right leg amputated below the knee 15 years before the study, and now has a swollen painful left leg. The spin echo image (Figure 3.12a shows a smaller artery to the amputated limb and an abnormality of the iliac vein. The field even echo rephasing magnitude image (Figure 3.12b) shows that the artery to the amputated limb is smaller and there is obstruction in the vein. Collateral veins also show on the side with venous obstruction. The velocity map, in which white shows blood flowing away from the heart and grey to black shows blood flowing towards the heart (Figure 3.12c) shows that the velocity in the smaller artery to the limb which was amputated is identical with the velocity in the normal leg. The areas under the curve, however, indicate a differential total flow. The velocity profiles in the veins show normal plug flow on the right and a higher velocity in the partially obstructed vein on the left, with a spike of very high velocity on one surface of the vein which is probably fast enough to scour away prostacyclin, endothelial derived relaxation factor, and other protective elements, thereby making this into a self-propagating disease by allowing continued deposition of platelets and the secretion of platelet derived growth factor.

It is of little value, however, merely to visualize plaques. What is needed is a method of determining whether the disease is active. This can be done using the property of nuclear magnetic resonance known as chemical shift. The proton in water precesses more freely and faster than it does when locked into a lipid. By detecting the signal at the water or fat frequencies, images can be produced which highlight

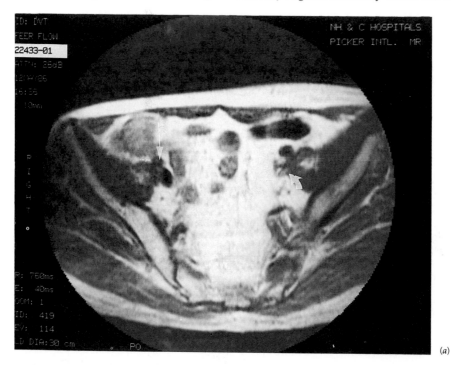

(a)

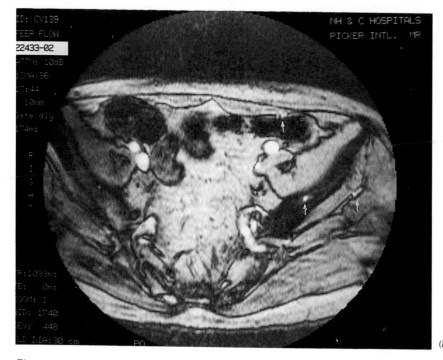

(b)

Figure 3.12

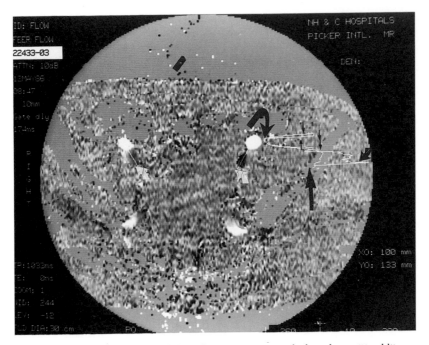

Figure 3.12 (*a*) A cross-section of the pelvis in a patient with thromboangitis obliterans migrans (Berger's disease) who still smokes. The right leg was amputated below the knee 15 years before this study. The right leg iliac artery (straight arrow) is smaller than the normal one on the left. The left iliac vein is abnormal (curved arrow). (*b*) The field even echo re-phasing (FEER) magnitude image corresponding with (*a*). The inferior epigastric veins and obturator veins and other small collateral veins are dilated (arrowed). (*c*) The phase map corresponding to the spin-echo image (*a*) and the FEER magnitude image (*b*). Velocity profiles have been produced across the iliac veins and arteries on both sides (curved white arrows). The large black arrow indicates the base line, to the left of which are the velocity profiles in the normal left iliac artery (upper small black arrow) and the small iliac artery (lower small black arrow). The peak velocities in the two vessels are identical (curved black arrow). If a limb is amputated, the artery becomes smaller and the blood velocity remains constant. The venous velocities do not correspond. The flow in the normal vein is indicated by the double black arrow, whereas the higher velocity in the abnormal vein is indicated by the curved black arrow, suggesting a spike of high velocity in the occluded vein with sufficient velocity to scour away protective prostacyclin, endothelial derived relaxation factor (EDRF) and other protective agents

water or fat whilst suppressing the other. If both images are produced of the same region and subtracted, the mixture of lipid and water can be determined. Atheroma contains up to 28% lipid, and concentrations of 0–30% fall on the straight-line part of the subtraction graph shown in Figure 3.13. Figure 3.14(a) shows an atheromatous plaque with a high signal and the corresponding histology; Figure 3.14(b) shows a high concentration of lipid. Figure 3.14(c) shows a plaque with no signal and the corresponding histology. Figure 3.14(d) shows absence of lipid. Figure 3.14(e) shows an aorta with obvious plaque. Figure 3.14(f) shows the eccentric plaque and, in Figure 3.14(g), the low signal on the subtraction image shows this to be a fibrous plaque. In Figure 3.14(h) an atheromatous plaque is seen and in Figure 3.14(i) the subtraction image shows high signal. This is a lipid-rich active plaque which is amenable to treatment. This technique does not image crystalline lipid. Any lipid seen on a

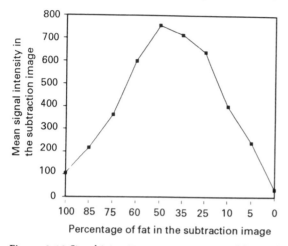

Figure 3.13 Signal intensity versus percentage of fat produced by floating oil on water in a tube and taking images with the slice incorporating various percentages of the fat. Atheroma containing 0–28% of lipid corresponds with the staight-line part of the graph on the right

subtraction image, therefore, is in the liquid phase and at risk of ulceration, surface thrombosis, and so on.

The coronary circulation

Another method of gaining information about the status of the coronary arteries is to study the back flow in the root of the aorta. In the normal aorta, whatever the compliance, there is a standard sequence of events following ventricular ejection. At first, as the aortic valve opens, there is 'plug' flow with a very flat velocity profile. This changes rapidly to a more normal profile of velocity but, due to the curvature of the aorta, this rapidly becomes asymmetric. After about 200 ms of systole, the asymmetry develops to form an internal circulation with some blood flowing backwards towards the root of the aorta which is destined for the coronary arteries. In the normal, this backflow divides into two streams, corresponding to flow in the two sinuses of Valsalver which contain the coronary arteries. If one coronary artery is partially occluded, the pattern of backflow is disturbed and the flow towards the relevant coronary sinus is diminished[8].

For the early detection of coronary arterial disease, monitoring the efficacy of preventive and therapeutic measures is vital; and for the management of patients with occlusion, visualization of the coronary arteries and measurement of flow in them is vital. The coronary arteries can be seen in transverse, vertical long axis, horizontal long axis and short axis images. The quality of the image of the coronary arteries, however, is degraded by misregistration of the heart from beat to beat. Nevertheless, credible mapping of velocity can often be achieved. Visualization of a coronary artery is not adequate to show its patency, although many publications exist suggesting this to be the case. Flow is easier to measure in coronary vein grafts than it is in the coronary arteries, although, as described below, measurements of

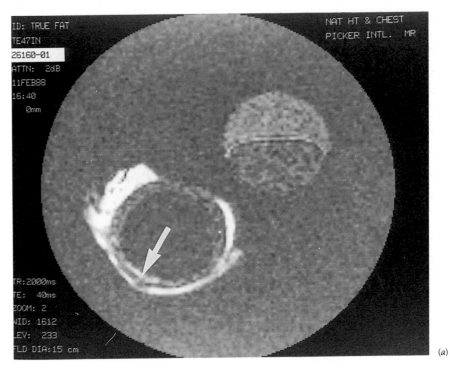

(a)

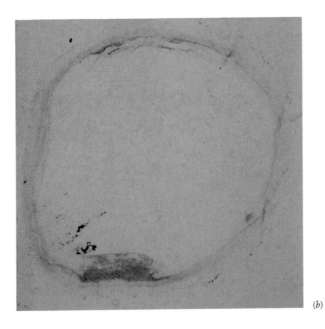

(b)

Figure 3.14

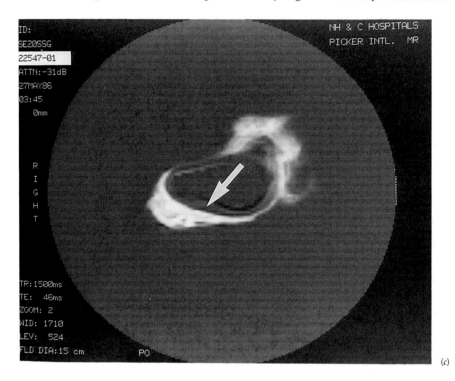

(c)

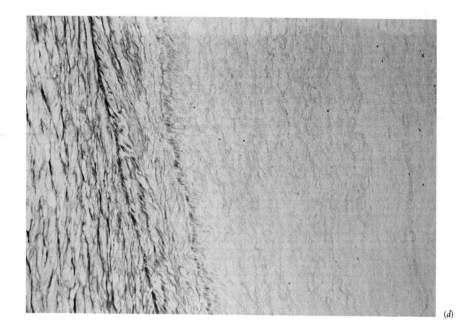

(d)

Figure 3.14

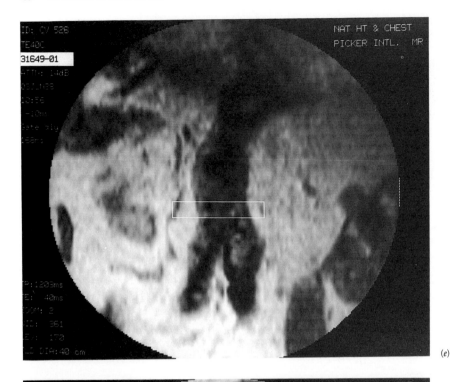

(e)

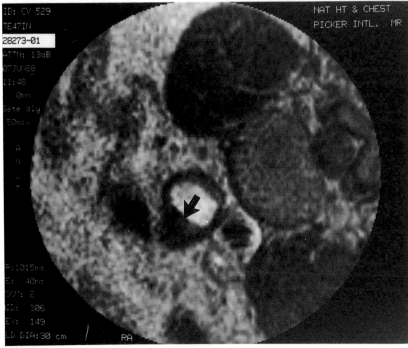

(f)

Figure 3.14

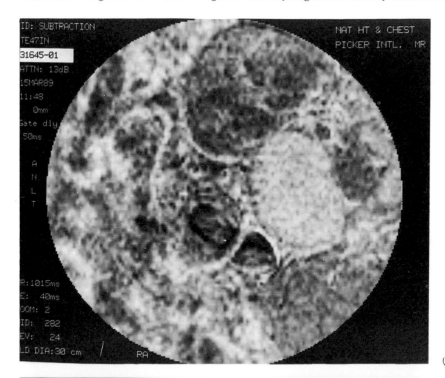

(g)

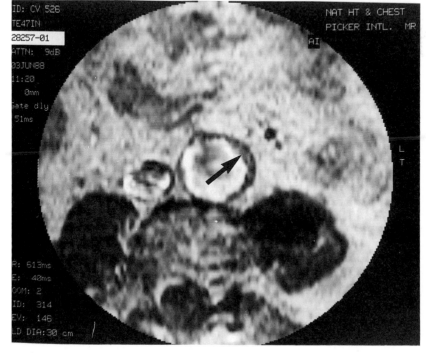

(h)

Figure 3.14

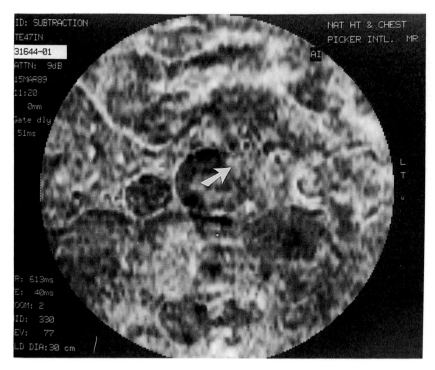

(i)

Figure 3.14 (*a*) A cross-section of a cadaver aorta. The subtraction image shows high signal in the plaque (arrowed) and the corresponding histological section, confirm this. (*b*) The corresponding histology to (*a*) stained with orange-red oil to highlight fat. This confirms a high concentration of lipid. (*c*) A plaque (arrowed) with low signal in the subtaction image, suggesting the absence of lipid. (*d*) An elastic Van Giessen stain showing absence of lipid corresponding with the subtraction image in (*c*). (*e*) An aorta with obvious plaque. The site of the cross-section image in (*b*) is indicated. (*f*) A spin-echo image corresponding to (*e*). The eccentric plaque (arrowed) can be seen. (*g*) The subtraction image corresponding to (*f*). There is low signal, confirming that this is a fibrous plaque not amenable to treatment. (*h*) A young patient with a plaque (arrowed). (*i*) The subtraction image showing high signal in the plaque, showing that this is a lipid-rich active plaque amenable to treatment

coronary flow can be clinically useful. Figure 3.15(a) is a spin-echo image showing two coronary vein grafts in a patient whose history and other studies suggest inadequacy of the graft to the territory of the right coronary artery. This is not indicated on the spin-echo image, in which the flow void is well seen. Every surgeon, however, is aware of the graft in which there is pulsitility but, due to poor run-off, the flow through the graft is inadequate. Figure 3.15(b) is the field even echo re-phasing magnitude image in the same patient and Figure 3.15(c) the corresponding velocity map. From measurement of velocities at various times throughout the cardiac cycle, it can be seen that there is nearly 2 ml of blood flowing through the graft in each cardiac cycle, whereas there is no measureable flow in the graft on the right. This cautionary tale applies also to the native coronary arteries. Figure 3.16(a) is a horizontal long axis image showing the right and left coronary arteries. Figure 3.16(b) is the corresponding field even echo re-phasing magnitude image and Figure 3.16(c) the velocity map showing that the velocity in the right and left coronaries

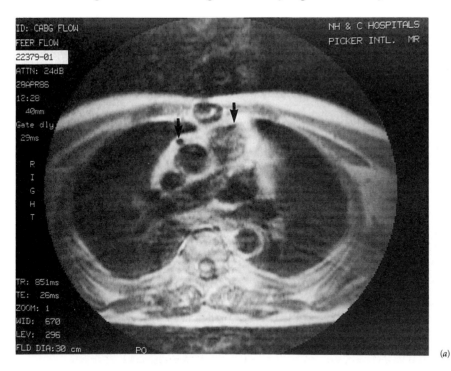

(a)

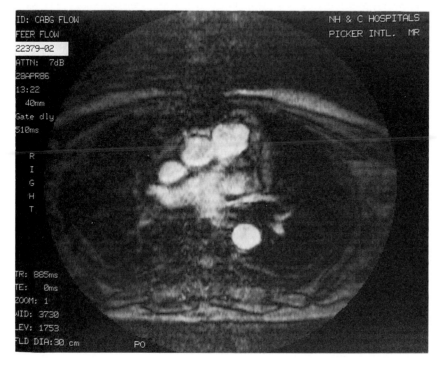

(b)

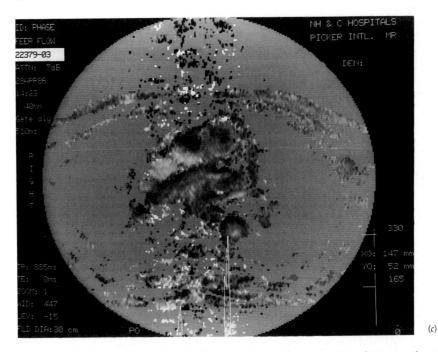

(c)

Figure 3.15 (*a*) A spin-echo image of a patient with two coronary vein grafts (arrowed), with a history suggesting that the graft to the right coronary artery territory is unsatisfactory. The two grafts both appear patent (arrowed). (*b*) The field even echo re-phasing magnitude image corresponding to (*a*) showing the presence of plaque in both coronary vein grafts. (*c*) The velocity map corresponding to (*a*) and (*b*). The velocity profiles show that there is good flow in the graft to the left territory with nearly 2 ml of blood flowing through the graft in each cardiac cycle and there is virtually no measurable flow on the right. This series of illustrations shows that the presence of a flow void on a spin-echo image does not indicate a patent graft

obeys the rule that the velocities in paired vessels are similar unless there is an obstruction. Figure 3.16(d) is the field echo re-phasing magnitude image in a patient who at angiography was thought to have narrowing of the anterior descending vessel. Figure 3.16(e) shows a series of velocity profiles along the length of the vessel, showing that there is no speeding up of blood past an obstruction and no stenosis is present.

Rapid imaging

There are several rapid imaging techniques, including fast low-angle shots and echo planar which produce good cardiac images. Images obtained with fast low-angle shots, however, take up to 100 m/s to acquire and are not appropriate for coronary vessels. Echo planar images, in contrast, can be acquired in less than 32 m/s with velocity encoding[14]. When these techniques are fully developed, they may allow reliable assessment of coronary flow.

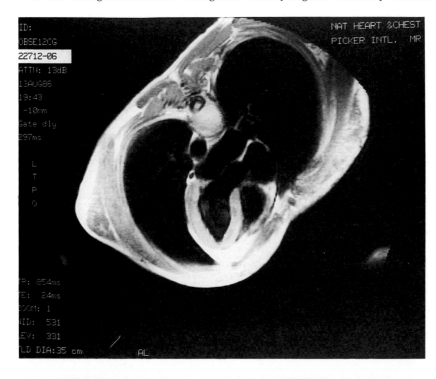

(a)

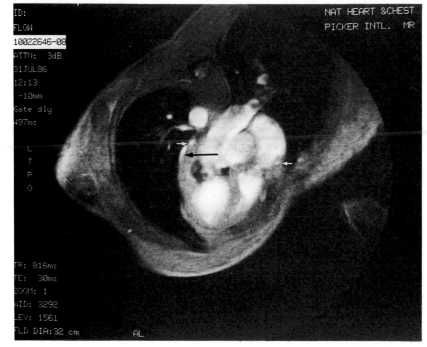

(b)

Figure 3.16

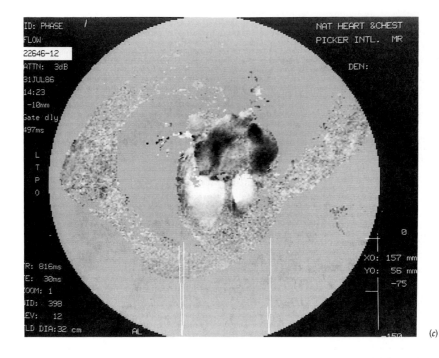

(c)

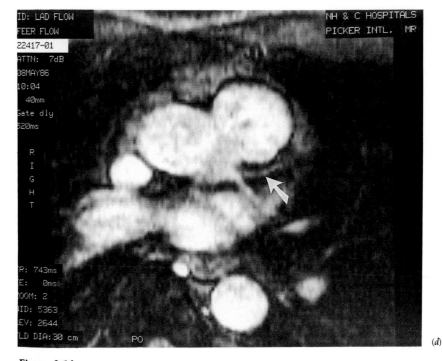

(d)

Figure 3.16

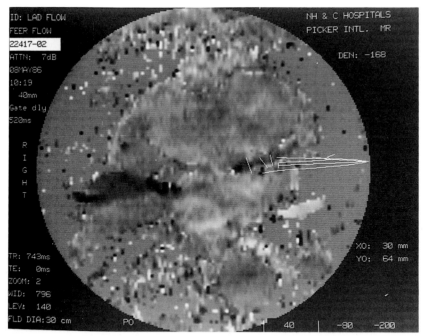

ID: LAD FLOW
FEER FLOW
22417-02
ATTN: 7dB
08MAY86
10:19
   40mm
Gate dly
520ms

R
I
G
H
T

TR: 743ms
TE: 0ms
ZOOM: 2
WID: 796
LEV: 140
FLD DIA:30 cm

NH & C HOSPITALS
PICKER INTL. MR

DEN: -168

XO: 30 mm
YO: 64 mm

PO   40   -80 -200   (e)

Figure 3.16 (a) A horizontal long axis in which the right and left coronary arteries can be seen in the corresponding atrioventricular grooves. (b) The field even echo re-phasing (FEER) magnitude image corresponding to (a). The right and left coronary arteries are arrowed in white and the tail of the coronary sinus is arrowed in black. (c) The corresponding velocity map showing approximately the same velocities in the right and left coronary arteries in this normal subject. (d) A FEER magnitude image in a patient who at angiography was suspected of having an occlusion in the left anterior descending artery, arrowed. This was somewhat improbable because of the patient's history and was more likely to be spasm, which was confirmed by velocity mapping, shown in (e). (e) A series of velocity profiles along the anterior descending coronary artery. These are taken at random and show the velocity to be independent of position, indicating that there is no occlusion, otherwise there would have to be an increase in velocity

Myocardial perfusion (using contrast agents)

A bolus injection of contrast agent, combined with acquisition using cine-magnetic resonance with the appropriate sequence, can be used to assess myocardial perfusion. At the moment, however, this requires a number of acquisitions using separate slices to assess the perfusion of the whole of the myocardium. This makes it a time-consuming process, requiring several injections of medium. One-shot imaging promises to make the use of contrast medium in mapping perfusion a viable method of study.

The role of contrast agents in magnetic resonance of the heart is not properly established. Suitable agents will undoubtedly be vital for the study of diffusion/perfusion of the myocardium, and for studying distribution of blood dynamically. It has to be borne in mind, however, that sequences of magnetic resonance can be devised to highlight movement and acceleration or still materials. Those radiologists who like the concept of contrast agents may not be in charge of cardiovascular diagnosis using magnetic resonance, in which case the role of specific contrast agents will be essential but their widespread use may be much more restricted.

Availability of magnetic resonance

Unfortunately, machines demonstrating magnetic resonance are still expensive, user-unfriendly and confining for the patient because they use a large solenoid magnet. At present, they are unsuitable for the assessment of the acutely ill. Their slowness at present makes the study of the coronary circulation unreliable. Most of the present generation of machines are refinements based on the first commercial machine made by EMI (still in use at the Hammersmith Hospital). These machines all use xy reconstruction which needs a minimum of 64 acquisitions. When gated to the heartbeat, this process takes a considerable time. Unlike this original machine, which operates at 0.15 tesla, most machines work at much higher field strengths where the motional artefact becomes a problem. Rooms shielded for radio frequency signals are necessary which, combined with the costly high-field magnets, makes the equipment very expensive. Recent developments include low-cost open-access magnets, the abandonment of powerful mini-computers in favour of processing distributed amongst dedicated immensely powerful boards, and better sequences (including rapid imaging) to increase the throughput of patients. Machines for cardiovascular magnetic resonance will shortly no longer be comparable in cost with positron emission tomography, the cardiac catheter laboratory and high-speed computerized tomography, but will cost in the region of twice a colour Doppler ultrasound machine (approximately the same as low-cost computerized tomography). This reduction in cost, along with increased efficiency combined with the public disquiet about irradiation, all suggest that magnetic resonance will become the workhorse diagnostic instrument of choice in the future.

Conclusion

Magnetic resonance can already contribute to the management of established coronary arterial disease. Images may show areas of abnormal myocardium which can be highlighted with the use of pharmacological stress. The reserve for coronary arterial flow can be assessed by measuring coronary sinus flow before and after the administration of coronary arterial vasodilators. Techniques are being developed that may be clinically useful in measuring coronary arterial flow directly. The real contribution to the continuum of management of coronary disease, however, hopefully lies in its preventive potential. Already aortic compliance, and velocity of pulse waves suggest a method of screening to detect arteriopaths. Already in patients with atheromatous plaques detected outside the coronary circulation, it has been possible to measure the plaques accurately, to determine their haemodynamic significance and to measure their content of lipid relevant to the breakdown of plaques causing acute events. Hopefully, discussion of the cardiological continuum in a few years time will shift their emphasis away from the management of end-state disease towards early detection and monitoring the efficacy of preventive and therapeutic measures. The ambition of cardiologists should be to allow people to live a normal lifespan without the quality of the end of their lives being diminished by the effects of occlusive vascular disease, as was so beautifully described by the poet Dryden over 300 years ago:

'Of no distemper, of no blast he died,
but fell like autumn-fruit that mellowed long,
Ev'n wondered at because he dropp'd no sooner,
Fate seemed to wind him up for four score years
Yet freely ran he on ten winters more;
Til, like a clock worn out with eating time,
The weary wheels of life at last stood still.'

Acknowledgements

I thank my colleagues, the Board of Governors of the National Heart & Chest Hospitals and the National Heart & Lung Institute, the Coronary Artery Disease Research Association Charity (CORDA) which has funded most of this work, and the Medical Research Council.

Appendix

The principles of nuclear magnetic resonance (NMR)

NMR is sometimes termed MRI, standing for magnetic resonance imaging. This does not take into account functional or biochemical measurements made using magnetic resonance spectroscopy and chemical shift imaging, therefore in this chapter the more accurate descriptive terms, magnetic resonance and nuclear magnetic resonance, are used.

The simplest atom is the hydrogen atom which consists of one positively charged particle − a proton − which forms the nucleus and one negatively charged electron loosely associated with it moving at nearly the speed of light. More complicated nuclei contain more than one proton and some also contain additional particles − neutrons − which are made up of combined protons and electrons.

Protons are abundant in the hydrogen in body water, body fat, electrolytes and organic chemicals. The work described in this chapter is based on proton resonance, though the nuclei of the atoms of some other elements contain a single, positive electric charge and can be studied by nuclear magnetic resonance.

Atomic nuclei spin on their axes at about a billion billion revolutions per minute. Spinning charges on the protons (and other nuclei which also have a lone, positive charge) create tiny magnetic fields just as an electric current passing round a coil of wire generates a magnetic field.

Magnetic nuclei in the body (and all matter) tend to line up in the earth's magnetic field. Unlike familiar compass needles which always line up with the north-seeking pole pointing north and the south-seeking pole south, atomic nuclei line up in almost equal numbers parallel with the magnetic field and the wrong way round, anti-parallel with the field. The ratio of nuclei lined the correct way round, increases with magnet field strength.

At 0.5 tesla, a commonly used field strength, about six in a million more lie the correct way round than anti-parallel. At 1.5 tesla, another common imaging field strength, this increases to about 10 in a million (1 tesla = 10 000 gauss; the earth's magnetic field varies between 0.3 and 0.7 gauss).

An object that is spinning in a field and that is perturbed will wobble about its axis of spin and precess at a much lower rate than its spin. A child's top spinning at several thousand rpm will precess through an apparently infinite number of angles at a few rpm. Protons precess at a frequency that is related to the strength of the magnetic field; the stronger the field the faster they precess. The radio frequency that corresponds to a particular field strength for a nucleus is known as the resonant frequency, or the Larmor frequency, for that nucleus.

The spinning proton in a typical clinical imaging magnet precesses at between 21 million and 65 million times per second (see resonant frequency below).

The smallest amount of energy available to perturb a proton to make it precess is one quantum which is large in comparison with the mass of a proton. One quantum of energy will cause a proton to precess at an angle of 54°. Application of a further quantum of energy will transfer the proton from the low-energy (parallel) state to the high-energy state (anti-parallel).

Precessing atomic nuclei possessing an electric charge will induce a voltage in a radio receiver aerial at radio frequencies corresponding to the rate of precession. All matter, including protons in the body, emit radio noise but, since nuclei do not precess in unison, this radio noise is detected as a random hiss.

Production of an image

Several steps have to be taken to produce an image from precessing protons.

The patient is placed in a strong magnetic field to align the nuclei. The axis of the field is known as the Z axis.

A radio frequency pulse applied at the resonant frequency, rotating round the long axis of the magnet, will cause energy to be absorbed and a number of parallel nuclei to become anti-parallel. When the radio frequency pulse is turned off, they return to the resting state with a time constant known at T1.

Slice selection – The property of the resonant frequency is used to obtain spatial resolution. The machine used for magnetic resonance is constructed with three sets of supplementary magnet coils which can create magnetic gradients in three orthogonal planes. (These are not necessarily parallel to the axis of the main magnet, known as the Z axis, enabling compound oblique imaging.) A gradient is applied perpendicular to the plane which is to be selected for imaging. A radio frequency pulse is applied to resonate with protons in a slice where the magnetic field strength corresponds to the resonant frequency. The wider the bandwidth of the radio frequency pulse, the thicker the slice. Most images use a slice which is 10 mm or less in thickness. The best cardiovascular images are usually produced using a slice 3 mm thick or less.

Spacial resolution in the slice – After slice selection, a radio receiver will detect a signal at the resonant frequency of the protons in the slice. This signal contains information about the total number of protons present in the slice but there is no spatial information within the signals. Two further gradients, known as the phase encoding and the read gradients, are then required at right angles to the slice selection gradient and to each other. These orthogonal planes are relayed to the Z axis and are known as the X and Y planes.

The read gradient – A magnetic gradient applied perpendicularly to the slice selection gradient in the X axis causes protons on the side of the slice experiencing the stronger field to precess faster and those on the weaker side to precess slower. A receiver capable of detecting all the frequencies emanating from the slice will detect a humble of radio noise. A Fourier transformation, which gives a spectrum of power related to frequency, of this signal will give spatial information in the axis of the gradient. A signal at a certain frequency emanates from the plane in the slice where the resonant frequency corresponds with the field strength. The amplitude of the signal relates to the number of protons present. Gradients and a Fourier transformation are also necessary to obtain spatial and volume information in the second axis.

The phase encoding gradient – The phase encoding gradient is used to obtain spatial resolution in the second direction. A gradient applied in the Y axis will cause the frequency in the low magnetic field to diminish and in the high field to increase. This gradient is applied for each radio frequency stimulation at a different strength or for a different period of time, affecting the phase change across the patient differently. A zero phase encoding gradient allows the phase to remain constant across the patient. A small gradient will cause a small phase shift or 'signature'. A stronger gradient will cause a larger shift. Usually, 64 or more phase encoding gradients are used and a slow Fourier transform enables spatial resolution in the axis perpendicular to the read gradient.

Spin echo – After the initial 180° RF pulse, which is used to put energy into the system and reverse the orientation of the protons, a second 90° radio frequency pulse is used to bring the nuclei into phase to produce a coherent signal. Because nuclei in different magnetic field strengths precess at different frequencies, local magnetic field differences soon dephase the protons which have been brought into phase to give a coherent signal. Local field differences are due to the local chemical environment and to small inhomogeneities in the main magnet due to imperfect manufacture and to the magnetic effects of the patient. The combination of these inhomogeneities produces a dephasing with a time constant known as T2. If the magnetic field is reversed, or if a further 180° radio frequency pulse is applied to invert the protons, the same inhomogeneities that caused dephasing will rephase the nuclei and a second and multiple signals can be obtained. These are known as spin echoes. In normal imaging, the phase-encoding gradient is applied once per heartbeat and the image is built up over a period of time, usually involving 64 or 128 heartbeats.

Echo planar – For rapid imaging, the gradients may be changed as frequently as every millisecond a whole image produced in 64 m/s.

Velocity encoding – Velocity and acceleration can be encoded in the MR signal in both conventional, slow imaging and echo planar imaging by using special techniques which encode movement as a change in the phase of the radio signal. The field even echo re-phasing (FEER) method was developed in the Magnetic Resonance Unit of the Royal Brompton National Heart and Lung Hospital and is the standard method of measuring velocity or acceleration accurately.

References

1. *Lancet*. Brain damage after open heart surgery. *Lancet*, **i**, 1161–1163, 1983
2. Longmore, D.B. The principles of magnetic resonance. *Br. Med. Bull.*, **45**, 848–880, 1989
3. Pennell, D.J., Underwood, S.R. and Longmore, D.B. Detection of coronary artery disease using MR imaging with dipyridamole infusion. *J. Comp. Asst. Tomogr.*, **14**, 167–170, 1990
4. Nayler, G.L., Firmin, D.N. and Longmore, D.B. Blood flow imaging by cine magnetic resonance. *J. Comp. Asst. Tomogr.*, **10**, 715–722, 1986

5. Firmin, D.N., Kilner, P.J., Pennell, D.J., et al. Short Echo Time (3.5–6 ms) Field Even Echo Rephasing Sequences for Improved Accuracy and Reliability of Blood Flow Velocity and Acceleration Measurements, vol. 8, Society of Magnetic Resonance in Medicine, Berkeley, p. 888 (Abstract), 1989

6. Klipstein, R.H., Firmin, D.N., Underwood, S.R., et al. Blood flow patterns in the human aorta studied by magnetic resonance. Br. Heart J., 58, 316–323, 1987

7. Bogren, H.G., Klipstein, R.H., Firmin, D.N. et al. Quantitation of antegrade and retrograde blood flow in the human aorta by magnetic resonance velocity mapping. Am. Heart J., 117, 1214–1222, 1989

8. Bogren, H.G., Klipstein, R.H., Firmin, D.N. et al. Ante and Retrograde Aortic Blood Flow in Normal Subjects and in Patients with Coronary Artery Disease Studied by Magnetic Resonance. Association of University Radiologists, New Orleans, 1988

9. Bogren, H.G., Mohiaddin, R.H., Klipstein, R.H., et al. The function of the aorta in ischemic heart disease: a magnetic resonance and angiographic study of aortic compliance and blood flow patterns. Am. Heart J., 118, 234–247, 1989

10. Mohiaddin, R.H., Underwood, S.R., Bogren, H.G., et al. Regional aortic compliance studied by magnetic resonance imaging: the effects of age, training and coronary artery disease. Br. Heart J., 62, 90–96, 1989

11. Bogren, H.G., Klipstein, R.H., Mohiaddin, R.H., et al. Pulmonary artery distensibility and blood flow patterns: a magnetic resonance study of normal subjects and of patients with pulmonary hypertension. Am. Heart J., 118, 990–999, 1989

12. Mohiaddin, R.H., Firmin, D.N., Underwood, S.R., et al. Chemical shift magnetic resonance imaging of human atheroma. Br. Heart J., 62, 81–89, 1989

13. Mohiaddin, R.H. and Longmore, D.B. MRI studies of atherosclerotic vascular disease: structural evaluation and physiological measurements. Br. Med. Bull., 45, 968–990, 1989

14. Firmin, D.N., Klipstein, R.H., Hounsfield, G.N., et al., Echo-planar high-resolution flow velocity mapping. Mag. Res. Med., 12, 316–327, 1989

4

Silent ischaemia – iceberg or mirage?

David Mulcahy and Kim Fox

Introduction

For many years, the investigation and reporting of coronary arterial disease was based on the study of patients who presented with symptoms of angina pectoris or acute myocardial infarction. Medical treatment was devised to reduce symptoms and, hopefully, result in a reduction in the risk of acute myocardial infarction and sudden death. The primary end-point of coronary arterial bypass surgery and, more latterly, of percutaneous transluminal coronary angioplasty, was to improve quality of life in patients with restrictive symptoms of angina, and hopefully to improve survival. 'Symptoms' was the password to investigation and treatment. Reports did appear in the literature about 'Coronary thrombosis without pain'[1] while observers noted that changes in the ST segment could occur in the absence of angina[2]. This was referred to by Paul Wood as 'latent angina'[2]. It was also known that sudden cardiac death could occur without warning[3]. Although these studies suggested that ischaemic heart disease could occur without any warning symptoms, it was not until the introduction of ambulatory monitoring of the ST segment as a research tool that the concept of silent but active ischaemic heart disease was glamourized. Thus, in 1974 Stern and Tzivoni[4] reported that many patients with coronary arterial disease have episodes of asymptomatic depression of the ST segment during their daily lives. This observation was, subsequently, confirmed by many authors[5,6], who noted that the majority of episodes of change in the ST segment in populations with coronary arterial disease occur without symptoms. Added interest in active but asymptomatic coronary arterial disease came with the report by Kannel[7] that approximately 15% of all acute myocardial infarctions were silent. Various researchers suggested a 'cause and effect' relation between silent ischaemia and both silent myocardial infarction and sudden unheralded cardiac death. Soon word reached the media, and silent ischaemia was branded 'the silent killer'. Angina was now being referred to at medical symposia as 'the tip of the iceberg' of ischaemia.

So what is silent ischaemia? Is it the iceberg without the tip, or is it a mirage based on the criteria we have chosen electrocardiographically to represent ischaemia? Is silent ischaemia the silent killer? In this review, the subject of silent ischaemia will be critically appraised, with special emphasis based on the relation between silent ischaemia and both acute myocardial infarction and sudden cardiac death. We will also discuss whether available evidence suggests that we should alter our investigational practice to seek and treat silent ischaemia.

Silent ischaemia – the iceberg without the tip

Ischaemic change in patients with coronary arterial disease has been defined as more than 1 mm depression of the ST segment occurring 0.08 s after the J point and persisting for more than 1 minute during ambulatory monitoring, criteria previously used for diagnosing ischaemia during exercise testing. Using this definition, two facts become clear from studies using recording systems with a frequency response to record accurately the ST segment continuously. First, that many patients with stable angina pectoris have transient episodes of ischaemic change of the ST segment during their daily lives[4–6,8–10]. Second, that the majority of such episodes occur in the absence of symptoms[4–6,8–10]. In studies of patients with unstable angina, the same observations have been repeatedly made[11–13], as also in those studied following myocardial infarction[14,15]. Overall, it appears that approximately half of all patients with coronary arterial disease and either stable or unstable angina will have transient episodes of silent ischaemia, and between 60% and 90% of all transient ischaemic episodes recorded in such patient groups are not associated with angina. It seems reasonable, therefore, to conclude on the basis of available evidence that 'silent ischaemia is the iceberg without the tip'.

But does silent ST segment change represent true ischaemia, and are there any characteristic similarities between silent and painful ST segment change?

The evidence that silent ST segment change represents true ischaemia comes from various sources. The classic study from Deanfield et al., published in 1983[5] and using positron emmission tomography, confirmed that alterations in myocardial perfusion in association with depression of the ST segment were similar whether accompanied by symptoms or not. Levy et al.[16] showed that there were similar elevations in pulmonary arterial pressure during both silent and painful episodes of change in the ST segment. Rozanski et al.[17] demonstrated abnormalities of myocardial perfusion without symptoms which were equivalent to those associated with pain during mental stress exercises. Studies during percutaneous transluminal coronary angioplasty have reported significant changes of the ST segment in association with myocardial dysfunction during balloon inflation without angina[18,19] In addition to these reports, there are now many studies which show that standard anti-anginal medications significantly reduce the frequency of silent change of the ST segment[20–26], and that interventions such as bypass surgery[27] or coronary angioplasty[28] reduce or eradicate such episodes. Various reports have attempted to assess the differential characteristics of silent and painful ischaemia[29,30].

The overall conclusion is that, characteristically, silent and painful episodes of ischaemia are very similar in terms of heart rate at onset of ischaemia, increase in heart rate prior to ischaemia, duration of ischaemic episodes, and number of episodes not preceded by an increase in heart rate. We can surmise from this that 'silent ischaemia' is 'painful ischaemia without the pain'. But why is silent ischaemia silent? The simple answer is that we don't know! Many theories abound, including a defective anginal warning system[31], alterations in endorphin function[32], and a generalized defective perception of pain[33]. What is most striking, however, from the studies of silent ischaemia using ambulatory ST segment monitoring, is that the large majority of patients investigated for silent ischaemia will have presented with angina or symptomatic myocardial infarction. Furthermore, many patients with transient episodes of silent ischaemia will also have painful ischaemic episodes. Perhaps a more relevant question (again to which we do not have the answer) is why painful ischaemia is painful?

Silent ischaemia – the mirage

Two observations are worthy of mention when we attempt to explain why so much ischaemic change occurs in the absence of symptoms. The first applies to our method of assessment of silent ischaemia. When patients undergo ambulatory ST segment monitoring during daily life, they are asked to maintain detailed diaries and to record all symptoms at the time of occurrence. If patients, for any reason, do not record the occurrence of a symptom because they were indisposed, or because they felt it was not angina (a common remark), then all episodes of ST segment change occurring at these times will be classified as 'silent ischaemia'. This is particularly relevant in the morning hours of waking, the period of maximal ischaemic activity[34,35], when patients are likely to be busier and less inclined to record their symptoms. Meticulous recording of all symptoms would probably result in a significant reduction in the ratio of silent to painful ischaemic episodes. It would not, however, alter the overall frequency of ischaemia: that is, the total ischaemic burden would remain unchanged. The second point deserving of mention is that studies looking at the characteristics of silent and painful ischaemia[30] have noted that silent ischaemia tends to be associated with a lesser degree of depression of the ST segment. If the definition of ischaemic change was revised to depression greater than 2 mm, then more silent ischaemic episodes would probably be eliminated than painful ones. While this revision would undoubtedly reduce the sensitivity of any electrocardiographic test, it would also improve the specificity. Some episodes of change in the grey area of depression of the ST segment of 1 mm may probably be mediated by factors such as tachycardia, but not represent true ischaemia.

Overall evidence to date suggests that silent ischaemia is common in populations with coronary arterial disease, occurs significantly more frequently than painful ischaemia (although being charactieristically similar), and represents true ischaemia. On the basis of much research work over the past 15 years, we must conclude that silent ischaemia is not a mirage but a common event in the daily lives of many patients with ischaemic heart disease. We must, therefore, attempt to analyse the frequency and characteristics of silent ischaemia within subgroups of patients, the importance of such events in the development of the end-points of coronary arterial disease, and assess whether alternative approaches to investigation and treatment are warranted.

Frequency and characteristics of silent ischaemia

Studies using ambulatory monitoring of the ST segment in patients with stable angina pectoris have shown that between 33% and 50% will have silent ischaemia, depending on whether[9] (Figure 4.1) or not[10] (Figure 4.2) monitoring was performed while patients were not receiving anti-anginal therapy. Silent ischaemia occurs more frequently in patients with more severe coronary arterial disease[9,36] and in those with a positive exercise test for ischaemia[37–39]. Many authors have suggested that the pathophysiological mechanisms of ambulatory ischaemia differ from those causing ischaemia during formal exercise testing[5,8,40] because of differences in heart rates at the onset of ischaemia in the different settings. This has not been borne out in practice. One of the striking observations noted when comparing exercise testing and ambulatory monitoring of the ST segment is that those patients with silent (or painful) ischaemia during daily life almost invariably have a positive exercise test for ischaemia. More importantly, those with frequent

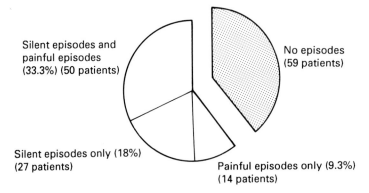

Silent episodes and
painful episodes
(33.3%) (50 patients)

No episodes
(59 patients)

Silent episodes only (18%)
(27 patients)

Painful episodes only (9.3%)
(14 patients)

Figure 4.1 Percentage frequency of painless and painful ischaemia during 6264 hours of ST segment monitoring in 150 unselected patients with coronary artery disease. (From reference 9, by permission.)

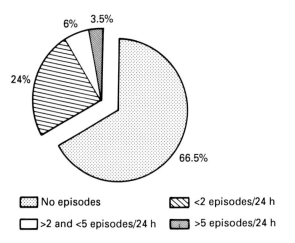

6%   3.5%

24%

66.5%

☒ No episodes   ☒ <2 episodes/24 h

☐ >2 and <5 episodes/24 h   ▨ >5 episodes/24 h

Figure 4.2 Frequency of episodes of silent ischaemia per 24 h in 114 patients on treatment. (From reference 10, by permission.)

daily episodes of silent ischaemia tend to have exercise tests which are positive at low work loads [37–39]. Patients with a negative exercise test rarely have significant ischaemia during their daily lives (Figure 4.3). This leads us to an important investigative conclusion: exercise testing, the standard electrocardiographic investigation for ischaemia, will identify those more likely to have ischaemia during their daily lives. By virtue of the fact that exercise testing is a more sensitive test in the diagnosis of coronary arterial disease [39], there is little indication, unless patients are unable to exercise, for the introduction of ambulatory monitoring for this purpose. Recent evidence suggests, none the less, that ambulatory monitoring may have an important part to play in stratification of risk in the patient with coronary arterial disease [41,42].

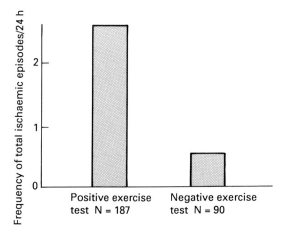

Figure 4.3 The relation between the mean frequency of total ischaemic episodes per 24 h on ambulatory electrocardiographic monitoring in patients with a positive and negative exercise test for ischaemia. (From reference 39, by permission.)

Prognosis in silent ischaemia

Recent evidence suggests that, within that group of patients with stable angina and a positive exercise test for ischaemia, additional evidence of ischaemia during daily life identifies a subgroup at increased risk of an adverse short- and medium-term outcome[41,42] (Figure 4.4). This has also been confirmed in studies of patients in the early and late stages following myocardial infarction[14,15] (Figure 4.5). One of the major areas of interest in silent ischaemia has related to the patient with unstable angina, one who is not suitable for exercise testing. Continuous monitoring of the ST segment in this group has shown silent ischaemia to be common[11–13], even after stabilization of symptoms, and to be associated with an adverse prognosis in short and medium term. These studies suggest that silent ischaemia is indeed important, that continuous monitoring of the ST segment offers prognostic information above and beyond that gleaned from the exercise test alone, and that its detection can help in stratification of risk in various subgroups of patients.

Silent ischaemia – the silent killer?: Relationship between silent ischaemia, acute myocardial infarction and sudden cardiac death

The prognostic studies quoted above imply that silent ischaemia may be the forerunner for unstable angina, myocardial infarction and sudden death, in addition to the rather softer end-points of requirement for coronary arterial bypass surgery and coronary angioplasty. Direct evidence for a cause-and-effect relation between silent ischaemia and both myocardial infarction and sudden death is, however, somewhat lacking to date, although indirect evidence abounds. Patients with silent ischaemia on exercise testing have been reported to be more likely to suffer myocardial infarction[43], and many patients resuscitated from ventricular fibrillation occurring out of hospital have been shown to have silent ischaemia on subsequent

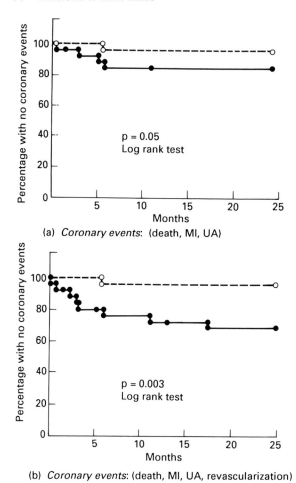

(a) *Coronary events*: (death, MI, UA)

(b) *Coronary events*: (death, MI, UA, revascularization)

Figure 4.4 Kaplan–Meier curves comparing the probability of (*a*) not experiencing an acute ischaemic event (death, myocardial infarction, unstable angina) and (*b*) progressive ischaemic event (acute events or revascularization for worsening symptoms) during follow-up for the 37 patients without ST segment depression (O---O) and the 49 patients with ST segment depression (●——●) as detected by ambulatory monitoring. MI = myocardial infarction; UA = unstable angina. (From reference 41, by permission.)

exercise testing[44]. Furthermore, there is a significant circadian variation of silent ischaemia[34,35], which corresponds with a similar pattern for acute myocardial infarction[45,46] and sudden cardiac death[47,48], with a peak in the morning waking hours (Figure 4.6).

Interestingly, beta-adrenergic blocking agents eradicate the morning peak of ischaemia[35], infarction[45] and sudden cardiac death[49] in a similar way, implying possibly similar pathophysiological mechanisms. This, of course, in no way implies that silent ischaemia directly leads to these end-points of cardiac disease, but simply suggests an association. It had been hoped that ambulatory monitoring would allow us to see 'live' the relationship between silent ischaemia and acute myocardial infarction and sudden cardiac death. What has been somewhat surprising is the low

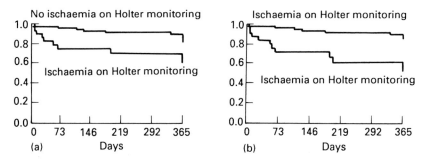

Figure 4.5 (*a*) Kaplan–Meier curves show probability of survival for 30 patients with and 73 patients without ST changes on Holter monitoring. Difference between probabilities for two groups is significant at P = 0.01 level (Peto test). (*b*) Kaplan–Meier curves show probability of survival without recurrent infarction for 30 patients with and 73 patients without ST changes on Holter monitoring. Difference between probabilities for two groups is significant at P = 0.001 level (Peto test). (From reference 14, by permission.)

frequency of ventricular arrhythmias associated with silent ischaemic episodes during daily life in patients with stable angina[9,50] and the relative paucity of documented sudden arrhythmic death or development of acute myocardial infarction in association with silent ischaemic change, despite the vast number of days of monitoring in patients with coronary arterial disease. A synopsis of the available prognostic studies and those looking specifically at the relation between silent ischaemia and the end-points of cardiac disease does not allow us to assume a cause-and-effect relationship. It may well be that silent ischaemia is only a marker of activity of disease, but does not lead to initiation of such events. This has important therapeutic implications as, although it is known that many anti-anginal agents significantly reduce the frequency of ambulatory ischaemia[20–26], there is relatively little hard evidence to suggest that these drugs benefit patients in terms of a reduction in the incidence of

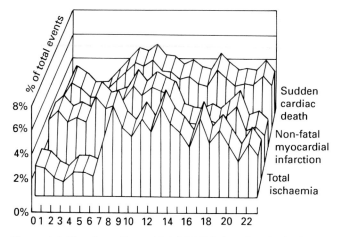

Figure 4.6 Circadian pattern of total (598) ischaemic episodes in our 150 patients when off therapy, of non-fatal myocardial infarction, and of sudden cardiac death. Plotted as percentage of total events during each hour of the day. (From reference 35, by permission.)

myocardial infarction and sudden death. There is little direct evidence, therefore, to justify at this time the title 'the silent killer' for silent ischaemia.

A new approach to management of the cardiac patient?

Much has been learnt over the past number of years about silent ischaemia. It is common and, in terms of significance, almost certainly equals that of ischaemia accompanied by pain. It is associated with an adverse prognosis in various subgroups of patients with coronary arterial disease. We must, therefore, reappraise our approach to the management of such patients. In subgroups with stable angina, and in those after infarction, an exercise test will identify those more likely to have ambulatory ischaemia. Monitoring of the ST segment in these may identify those patients at increased risk of an adverse outcome. At a time when waiting lists for intervention are ever increasing, stratification of risk using ambulatory monitoring in the presence of a positive exercise test may help in selecting those who are more likely to benefit from early intervention. The use of continuous monitoring of the ST segment in that population with unstable angina may be particularly rewarding, as it is clear that stabilization of symptoms does not necessarily lead to eradication of ischaemia. The identification of persisting silent ischaemia in these patients should point towards early investigation and treatment, thereby hopefully reducing the incidence of myocardial infarction and sudden death. In general, over the next decade it may be both necessary and rewarding to alter our management to treat the overall picture of ischaemia rather than base investigational and interventional decisions primarily on symptomatology. To take this expensive and invasive avenue of management we must satisfy ourselves that the identification and treatment of silent ischaemia, whether it be a marker or a direct catalyst for the end-points of coronary arterial disease, does indeed point towards a better outlook for the patient.

Conclusion

Silent ischaemia has been well characterized in populations with coronary arterial disease, and appears to be of prognostic significance, although a direct cause-and-effect link between it and the end-points of the disease remains tenuous. Much further research must be done to establish firmly whether the treatment of silent ischaemia is justified. From available evidence, a conclusion can be drawn that silent ischaemia is not a mirage, but represents the part of the iceberg that we cannot see, but of which we must be aware.

References

1. Boyd, L.D. and Werblow, S.C. Coronary thrombosis without pain. Am. J. Med. Sci., **194**, 814, 1937
2. Wood, P., McGregor, M., Magidson, O. and Whittaker, W. The effort test in angina pectoris. Br. Heart J., **12**, 363, 1950
3. Schatzkin, A., Cupples, L.A., Heeren, T., Morelock, S., Mucatel, M. and Kannel, W.B. The epidemiology of sudden unexpected death: risk factors for men and women in the Framingham Heart Study. Am. Heart J., **107**, 1300, 1984
4. Stern, S. and Tzivoni, D. Early detection of silent ischemic heart disease by 24 hour electrocardiographic monitoring of active subjects. Br. Heart J., **35**, 481, 1974

5. Deanfield, J.E., Maseri, A., Selwyn, A.P., *et al.* Myocardial ischaemia during daily life in patients with stable angina: its relation to symptoms and heart rate changes. *Lancet*, **ii**, 753, 1983

6. Cecchi, A.C., Dovellini, E.V., Marchi, F., *et al.* Silent myocardial ischemia during ambulatory electrocardiographic monitoring in patients with effort angina. *J. Am. Coll. Cardiol.*, **1**, 934, 1983

7. Kannel, W.B. and Abbott, R.D. Incidence and prognosis of unrecognised myocardial infarction. An update on the Framingham study. *N. Engl. J. Med.*, **311**, 1144, 1984

8. Schang, S.J. and Pepine, C.J. Transient asymptomatic S-T segment depression during daily activity. *Am. J. Cardiol.*, **39**, 396, 1977

9. Mulcahy, D., Keegan, J., Crean, P., *et al.* Silent myocardial ischaemia in chronic stable angina: a study of frequency and characteristics in 150 patients. *Br. Heart J.*, **60**, 417, 1988

10. Mulcahy, D., Keegan, J., Lindsay, D., *et al.* Silent myocardial ischaemia in patients referred for coronary artery bypass surgery because of angina: a comparison with patients whose symptoms were well controlled on medical treatment. *Br. Heart J.*, **61**, 496, 1989

11. Gottlieb, S.O., Weisfeldt, M.L., Ouyang, P., *et al.* Silent ischemia as a marker of early unfavorable outcomes in patients with unstable angina. *N. Engl. J. Med.*, **314**, 1214, 1986

12. Gottlieb, S.O., Weisfeldt, M.L., Ouyang, P., *et al.* Silent ischemia predicts infarction and death during 2-year follow-up of unstable angina. *J. Am. Coll. Cardiol.*, **10**, 756, 1987

13. Nademanee, K., Intarachot, V., Josephson, M.A., *et al.* Prognosis significance of silent myocardial ischemia in patients with unstable angina. *J. Am. Coll. Cardiol.*, **19**, 1, 1987

14. Gottlieb, S.O., Gottlieb, S.H., Achuff, S.C., *et al.* Silent ischemia on holter monitoring predicts mortality in high-risk post-infarction patients. *J. Am. Med. Assoc.*, **259**, 1030, 1988

15. Tzivoni, D., Gavish, A., Zin, D., *et al.* Prognostic significance of ischemic episodes in patients with previous myocardial infarction. *Am. J. Cardiol.*, **62**, 661, 1988

16. Levy, R.D., Shapiro, L.M., Wright, C. *et al.* The haemodynamic significance of asymptomatic ST segment depression assessed by ambulatory pulmonary artery pressure monitoring. *Br. Heart J.*, **56**, 526, 1986

17. Rozanski, A., Bairey, N., Krantz, D.S., *et al.* Mental stress and the induction of silent myocardial ischemia in patients with coronary artery disease. *N. Engl. J. Med.*, **318**, 1005, 1988

18. Sigwart, U., Grbic, M., Payot, M., *et al.* Ischemic events during coronary artery balloon occlusion. In *Silent Myocardial Ischemia* (eds. W. Rutishauser and H. Roskamm), Springer-Verlag, Berlin, pp. 29–36, 1984

19. Serruys, P.W., Wijns, W., van Brand, M., *et al.* Left ventricular performance, regional blood flow, wall motion and lactate metabolism during transluminal angioplasty. *Circulation*, **70**, 25, 1984

20. Uusitalo, A., Arstila, M., Bae, E.A., *et al.* Metoprolol, nifedipine, and combination in stable effort angina pectoris. *Am. J. Cardiol.*, **57**, 733, 1986

21. Quyyumi, A.A., Crake, T., Wright, C.M., *et al.* Medical treatment of patients with severe exertional and rest angina: double blind comparison of beta-blocker, calcium antagonist, and nitrate. *Br. Heart J.*, **8**, 124, 1987

22. Frishman, W.H. and Teicher, M. Antianginal drug therapy for silent myocardial ischemia. *Am. Heart J.*, **114**, 140, 1987

23. Imperi, G.A., Lambert, C.R., Coy, K., *et al.* Effects of titrated beta-blockade (metoprolol) on silent myocardial ischemia in ambulatory patients with coronary artery disease. *Am. J. Cardiol.*, **60**, 519, 1987

24. Frishman, W., Charlap, S., Kimmel, B., *et al.* Diltiazem, nifedipine, and their combination in patients with stable angina pectoris: effects on angina, exercise tolerance, and the ambulatory electrocardiographic ST segment. *Circulation*, **477**, 774, 1988

25. Egstrup, K. Randomised double blind comparison of metoprolol, nifedipine, and their combination in chronic stable angina: effects on total ischemic activity and heart rate at onset of ischemia. *Am. Heart J.*, **116**, 971, 1988

26. Cohn, P.F., Vetrovec, G.W., Nesto, R. and Gerber, F.R. The Nifedipine-Total Ischemia awareness program: A national survey of painful and painless myocardial ischemia including results of antiischemic therapy. *Am. J. Cardiol.*, **63**, 534, 1989

27. Quyyumi, A.A., Wright, C., Mockus, L., *et al.* Effects of myocardial revascularisation in patients with effort angina and those with effort and nocturnal angina. *Br. Heart J.*, **54**, 557, 1985

28. Josephson, M.A., Nademanee, K., Intarachot, V., *et al.* Abolition of holter monitor-detected silent myocardial ischemia after percutaneous transluminal coronary angioplasty. *J. Am. Coll. Cardiol.*, **10**, 499, 1987

29. Stern, S., Gavish, A., Weisz, G., *et al.* Characteristics of silent and symptomatic myocardial ischemia during daily activities. *Am. J. Cardiol.*, **61**, 1223, 1988

30. Mulcahy, D., Keegan, J. and Fox, K.M. Comparative characteristics of silent and painful ischaemia

during ambulatory ST segment monitoring in patients with coronary artery disease. *Int. J. Cardiol.*, **28**, 377, 1990.

31. Droste, C., Greenlee, M.W. and Roskamm, H. A defective anginal pectoris warning system: Experimental findings of ischemic and electrical pain test. *Pain*, **26**, 199, 1986
32. Ellestad, M.H. and Kuan, P. Naloxone and asymptomatic ischemia. Failure to induce angina during exercise testing. *Am. J. Cardiol.*, **54**, 928, 1984
33. Glazier, J.J., Chierchia, S., Brown, M.J. and Maseri, A.A. Importance of generalized defective perception of painful stimuli as a cause of silent myocardial ischemia in chronic stable angina pectoris. *Am. J. Cardiol.*, **58**, 667, 1986
34. Rocco, M.B., Barry, J., Campbell, S., *et al.* Circadian variation of transient myocardial ischemia in patients with coronary artery disease. *Circulation*, **75**, 395, 1987
35. Mulcahy, D., Keegan, J., Cunningham, D., *et al.* Circadian variation of total ischaemic burden and its alteration with antianginal agents. *Lancet*, **ii**, 755, 1988
36. Kunkes, S.H., Pichard, A.D., Smith, H., *et al.* Silent ST segment deviations and extent of coronary artery disease. *Am. Heart J.*, **100**, 813, 1980
37. Campbell, S., Barry, J., Rocco, M.B., *et al.* Features of the exercise test that reflect the activity of ischemic heart disease out of hospital. *Circulation*, **74**, 72, 1986
38. Epstein, S.E., Quyyumi, A.A. and Bonow, R.O. Current concepts: myocardial ischemia – silent or symptomatic. *N. Engl. J. Med.*, **318**, 1038, 1988
39. Mulcahy, D., Keegan, J., Sparrow, J., *et al.* Ischemia in the ambulatory setting – the total ischemic burden: Relation to exercise testing and investigative and therapeutic implications. *J. Am. Coll. Cardiol.*, **14**, 1166, 1989
40. Cohn, P.F. and Lawson, W.E. Characteristics of silent myocardial ischemia during out of hospital activities in asymptomatic angiographically documented coronary artery disease. *Am. J. Cardiol.*, **59**, 746, 1987
41. Rocco, M.B., Nabel, E.G., Campbell, S., *et al.* Prognostic importance of myocardial ischemia detected by ambulatory monitoring in patients with stable coronary artery disease. *Circulation*, **78**, 877, 1988
42. Deedwania, P., Carbajal, E., Nelson, J. and Linn, L. Silent ischemia during daily life is an independent predictor of survival in stable angina. *J. Am. Coll. Cardiol.*, **13**, 3A, 1989
43. Assey, M.E., Walters, G.L., Hendrix, G.H., *et al.* Incidence of acute myocardial infarction in patients with exercise-induced silent myocardial ischemia. *Am. J. Cardiol.*, **59**, 497, 1987
44. Sharma, B., Asinger, R., Francis, G.S., *et al.* Demonstration of exercise induced painless myocardial ischemia in survivors of out-of-hospital ventricular fibrillation. *Am. J. Cardiol.*, **59**, 740, 1987
45. Muller, J.E., Stone, P.H., Turi, Z.G., *et al.* Circadian variation in the frequency of onset of acute myocardial infarction. *N. Engl. J. Med.*, **313**, 1315, 1985
46. Hjalmarson, A., Gilpin, E.A., Nicod, P., *et al.* Differing circadian patterns of symptom onset in subgroups of patients with acute myocardial infarction. *Circulation*, **80**, 267, 1989
47. Muller, J.E., Ludmer, P.L., Willich, S.N., *et al.* Circadian variation in the frequency of sudden cardiac death. *Circulation*, **75**, 131, 1987
48. Willich, S.N., Levy, D., Rocco, M.B., *et al.* Circadian variation in the incidence of sudden cardiac death in the Framingham heart study population. *Am. J. Cardiol.*, **60**, 801, 1987
49. Peters, R.W., Muller, J.E., Goldstein, S., *et al.* Propranolol and the morning increase the frequency of sudden cardiac death (BHAT study). *Am. J. Cardiol.*, **63**, 1518, 1989
50. Quyyumi, A.A., Crake, T., Wright, C., *et al.* The incidence and morphology of ischaemic ventricular tachycardia. *Eur. Heart J.*, **7**, 1037, 1986

5

The clinical role of nuclear cardiology in assessing the myocardium at risk

Richard Underwood

Nuclear medicine has enjoyed a resurgence of interest in recent years as the value of the functional information that it provides is appreciated[1]. In almost every branch of medicine, radiopharmaceuticals are able to measure the function of organs and, combined with the anatomical information provided by other imaging techniques such as ultrasound and radiology, this allows a more objective approach to management of patients than when functional information is lacking. This review considers the way in which nuclear cardiology might influence the management of patients with coronary arterial disease, concentrating on its ability to assess the myocardium at risk in patients with stable angina, and also on technical developments which take nuclear medicine away from the days when the term 'unclear medicine' was, in some cases, justified.

Strategy of investigation in coronary arterial disease

To begin with an analogy: if conversation falters around the dinner table at a meeting concerned with magnetic resonance, a topic that can be guaranteed to revive interest is that of the optimum strength of the magnetic field. There is not, of course, a single answer to this question since it depends on the type of work that is anticipated. Those interested in spectroscopy or high-resolution images of small structures need a high field. Those interested in contrast between different tissues may prefer a lower field. And those interested in imaging a moving organ, such as the heart, may be happiest at intermediate fields. The debate is, in any case, academic except when choosing or installing a machine, and it will be eclipsed by the development of readily rampable magnets so that the strength of the field becomes just one of the many parameters that are optimized in an individual study. Until this happens, there is a simple, if cynical, answer: the optimum field strength is the one that you have.

The analogy can be transferred to other areas of clinical medicine. In cardiology, for instance, the best test for assessing a patient is the one that is readily available and with which the requesting physician is most familiar. This explains the widespread reliance of cardiologists on the coronary arteriogram when making management decisions in patients with coronary arterial disease. It cannot be denied that it is an effective tool. Of patients with stable angina, for instance, an analysis of data from the Framingham study[2] suggests that two-fifths undergo cardiac catheterization, and three-quarters of these have some form of mechanical intervention, either percutaneous transluminal coronary angioplasty or coronary arterial bypass grafting [3]. To put numbers to these proportions of patients in the USA, of 5 million people with stable angina or previous myocardial infarction, 2 million will undergo catheterization over a 5-year period and $1\frac{1}{2}$ million will have either angioplasty or surgery. Similar figures for Europe are difficult to estimate, but even allowing for a lower rate of catheterization and intervention, substantial numbers are involved. Thus, a large number of patients are well served by the traditional cardiological assessment of history, examination, exercise electrocardiography and coronary arteriography.

What, however, of the three-fifths of patients with stable angina who are not catheterized, one-fifth of whom will suffer myocardial infarction over a 5-year period? What of the large numbers of patients who present annually with myocardial infarction of sudden death [4]? Could this be avoided? Are we convinced that we are offering intervention to those who most need it? The solution to these difficult questions lies in some method of predicting the future: in other words, in the routine assessment of prognosis. It is in this area that nuclear medicine makes its most important contribution.

Hippocrates taught that the primary aim of a physician is to relieve symptoms and to do no harm. The cardiologist is most often concerned with the relief of angina. A stepped method of medical treatment followed by mechanical intervention in those with persistent symptoms is undoubtedly effective. If life were this simple, it could be argued that a history is the only test required, and the anatomical assessment of the coronary arteries would be performed only as a guide to the surgeon or interventional cardiologist. In practice, life is not this simple for two reasons. First, however skilled the taker of the history, and however lucid the patient, it is wise to have objective evidence of myocardial ischaemia before assuming that ischaemia is the cause of the patient's symptoms. Second, we now know that the extent of myocardial ischaemia is the most important prognostic indicator available. If we are able to measure this, we are able to do more than Hippocrates taught, since we can then employ available therapies in the hope of preventing future infarction and death.

Prognosis in coronary arterial disease

Prognosis in coronary arterial disease has long been known to depend upon the severity of the disease, but the problem lies in an objective assessment of severity. Many invasive cardiologists feel most at home if a coronary arteriogram is available. That there is a relationship between the severity of disease assessed in this way and the amount of myocardium in jeopardy is reflected in the better prognosis of patients with disease of the main stem of the left coronary artery, and three vessel disease, with surgical rather than medical treatment [5]. It must be accepted, however, that the coronary arteriogram is a very crude method of assessing the functional significance of disease. Visual assessment of coronary arteriograms has long been known to have a large variability both between and amongst observers [6,7] and to carry a poor association with anatomy as seen at autopsy [8–12]. More recently, a poor relationship has also been demonstrated between luminal narrowing and coronary arterial function [13]. Some attempt can be made to improve the assessment using either a coronary arterial score [14–16] or by digitizing tracings of the lesions to combine the effects of luminal narrowing and length and morphology of the stenosis [17]. The matter is complicated, however, by the fact that coronary arteries are not passive conduits but active organs [18] that control the shear stress along their walls by dilating in response to increases in flow[19]. This normal dilatation is impaired or reversed by atheromatous disease[20]. There can be no doubt, therefore, that the function of coronary arteries must be assessed by a separate technique, and that the main role of coronary arteriography is as an anatomical guide during angioplasty or surgery.

Of the functional tests, exercise electrocardiography is the one most widely performed. It is cheap, widely available, and it provides an objective assessment of the patient's symptoms under controlled conditions. Several parameters can provide prognostic information, including the time of exercise, the extent of depression of the ST segment, and the response of the blood pressure[21–24]. All of these, however, are crude measures of the presence of myocardial ischaemia. The time of exercise depends upon many factors, not all of which are related to the cardiovascular system, and the onset of angina is a relatively late phenomenon. Depression of the ST segment often occurs before angina, but it is, none the less, a relatively late indicator of ischaemia and it gives no information on the site or extent of ischaemia unless the relationship between depression of the segment and heart rate is examined[25–27]. The poor relationship between the site of ST segmental depression and the site of ischaemia is often forgotten. Many cardiologists mistakenly believe that they can distinguish between, say, disease of the left anterior descending or right coronary artery from the site of changes. In addition, changes in the ST segment are non-specific indicators of myocardial ischaemia, and interpretation is complicated by many factors including abnormalities at rest, drug therapy, and conduction defects. The response of the blood pressure requires a large area of myocardial ischaemia to be abnormal, and so it is a specific, but insensitive, indicator of a poor prognosis.

Nuclear cardiology in the assessment of prognosis

Radionuclide ventriculography

The other tests for assessing the function of the coronary arteries and predicting prognosis lie in the field of nuclear cardiology. Abnormalities of contraction can be seen at a relatively early stage in myocardial ischaemia and, hence, can be detected by radionuclide ventriculography (Plate 1). Extensive regional abnormalities will also impair global contraction, and this will be manifested in the left ventricular ejection fraction. The first report of exercise radionuclide ventriculography in patients with coronary arterial disease suggested a perfect separation between normal and diseased patients on the basis of the response of the ejection fraction[28]. If nothing else, the study illustrated the importance of selection of patients in determining sensitivity and specificity. Subsequent studies showed a more modest sensitivity[29–37]. Of course, there is no reason why perfect sensitivity of specificity should be expected, partly because of the dissociation between coronary arterial anatomy, and partly because only extensive myocardial ischaemia would be expected to lead to impaired global ventricular function. Earlier indicators of ischaemia might be abnormal timing of ventricular contraction manifested in the Fourier phase image[38] and, possibly, also diastolic function although this is more difficult to assess, especially during dynamic exercise[39].

Of greater clinical importance than mere detection of disease is the assessment of its significance and, hence, the risk of future events. Here, left ventricular ejection fraction is important[40–47]. But, should we measure the ejection fraction at rest or at exercise? Should we study the response to exercise, or one of many other parameters, such as end systolic volume or diastolic function? Measurement of the ejection fraction at rest certainly gives some prognostic information, but the ejection fraction during exercise appears to include this information and more. It does not matter whether the ejection fraction is low when stressed because it is low at rest, or because there is a large fall induced by the stress. In both cases, the risk is high for future events such as infarction and death. Thus, the important factor is the total amount of myocardium either infarcted or in jeopardy.

Myocardial perfusion imaging

If this is the case, perhaps it is most rational to look at myocardial perfusion directly, particularly as it is the earliest event in an episode of angina that can be detected simply. The evidence that imaging of myocardial perfusion by thallium-201 provides prognostic information in stable angina[48–53] and following myocardial infarction[54–58] is overwhelming. Even in asymptomatic patients, the thallium scan can identify those at high risk of future events[59,60]. The literature on the subject is too large to discuss in detail in this review, but two important papers are those from Ladenheim and colleagues[61,62]. In 1689 patients with coronary arterial disease without prior infarction, it was shown that the extent and the severity of the reversible defects detected using thallium-201 were independent predictors of cardiac events at one year[61]. The rate of cardiac events varied from 0.4% in patients with normal perfusion during exercise, to 78% in patients with both severe and extensive defects of perfusion. In a subsequent paper, the same group demonstrated the incremental prognostic power of the history, exercise electrocardiography, and imaging of myocardial perfusion[62].

Thus, it could be argued that imaging of myocardial perfusion should be performed in all patients with coronary arterial disease to assess prognosis and to select patients who, irrespective of symptoms, deserve intervention to prevent future infarction or death. Such a policy assumes that intervention can improve prognosis in patients with few or absent symptoms but large areas of reversible ischaemia. Although this has not been proved, there is some supporting evidence. It has been shown, for instance, that coronary angioplasty can be performed safely and with good anatomical results in asymptomatic patients with coronary arterial disease, and that the prognosis at 5 years is excellent[63]. Whether it is any better than without intervention remains to be established but, until this evidence is available, it is reasonable to assume that it is ultimately beneficial to abolish reversible ischaemia.

The powerful prognostic value of imaging of myocardial perfusion is slightly difficult to correlate with the increasing evidence that myocardial infarction need not occur by thrombosis on a severe stenosis. Lesions that do not limit flow may be equally active and thrombogenic. Little and colleagues[64] have shown that only one-third of infarctions occur because of occlusion of the most severe stenosis, and that two-thirds occur at stenoses that were less than 50%. Similar results have been shown by Hackett and colleagues[65] and by Brosius and Roberts[66]. Thus there will always be patients who present with myocardial infarction or sudden death without preceding angina. We do not yet have a diagnostic technique that is capable of detecting such early lesions. Presumably the prognostic power of the imaging of myocardial perfusion arises from the fact that patients with extensive lesions that limit flow are also likely to have thrombogenic lesions (even if not limiting flow) and, so, are at high risk of infarction.

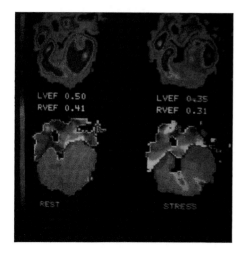

Plate 1 Amplitude (top) and phase images (bottom) reconstructed from equilibrium radionuclide ventriculography performed at rest (left) and during maximal dynamic exercise (right) in a patient with disease of a large left anterior descending coronary artery. Both left (LVEF) and right ventricular ejection fractions (RVEF) fall indicating stress-induced ischaemia. The amplitude and phase images show normal motion of both ventricles at rest. During stress there is hypokinesis (reduced amplitude) and delayed contraction (increased phase seen in yellow) affecting the septum and the apices of both ventricles

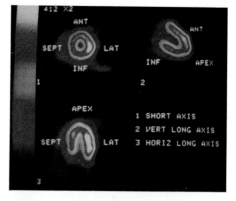

Plate 2 Thallium-201 emission tomograms in three perpendicular planes showing uniform uptake and, hence, normal perfusion throughout the myocardium

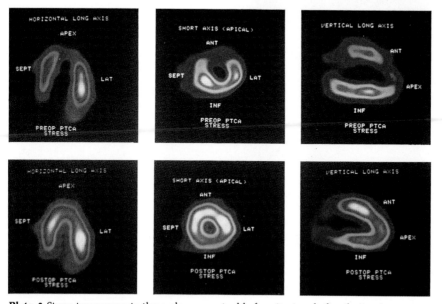

Plate 3 Stress tomograms in three planes acquired before (top) and after (bottom) angioplasty of a lesion in the left anterior descending artery. Before the procedure there is ischaemia of the distal anterior wall and apex with sparing of the septum. Afterwards, myocardial perfusion is normal

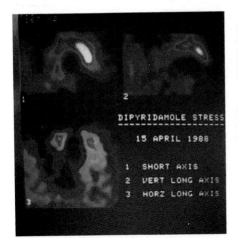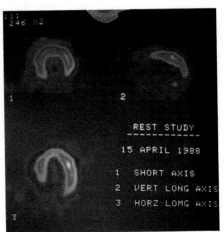

Plate 4 Stress (left) the redistribution (right) tomograms in a patient with severe coronary arterial disease. During stress there are extensive abnormalities with only a small region of the anterolateral wall normally perfused. Following redistribution, there is improvement in the septum and lateral walls but no change in the inferior wall. The patient had previous inferior infarction with an occluded right coronary artery and diseased left anterior descending and circumflex arteries. The normally perfused area was supplied by a good marginal branch of the left circumflex artery

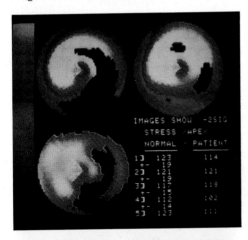

Plate 5 Stress (top left) and redistribution (top right) polar plots constructed from short axis thallium-201 tomograms of a patient with disease of the left circumflex coronary artery. The areas with abnormal uptake when compared with a normal population are blacked out. There is a defect of the lateral wall during stress which is much smaller at rest. The washout polar plot (bottom left) shows reduced washout from the abnormal area

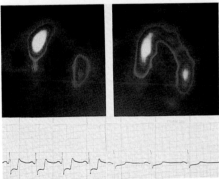

Plate 6 Immediate (left) and redistribution (right) horizontal long axis thallium-201 tomograms following intravenous infusion of dipyridamole without dynamic exercise. There is reversible ischaemia of the lateral wall which is also reflected in the electrocardiogram (lead CM5)

The limitations of thallium-201 scintigraphy

If thallium-201 scintigraphy is so valuable, why is it not used in all patients with coronary arterial disease? That it is underused has been demonstrated by a recent survey performed by the British Nuclear Cardiology Group[67]. The number of nuclear cardiological investigations performed in Great Britain in 1988 was 500 per million population. In the USA, the equivalent figure in 1985 was 3550[68]; but even there the use of nuclear cardiology is very patchy, with most studies being performed in a few active centres where other centres perform very few scans. These discrepancies highlight a number of problems with thallium-201 scintigraphy.

First, only 5% of the dose injected ends up in the myocardium, the remainder being taken up by skeletal muscle, stomach and gut. Second, the isotope has a relatively long half-life (72 h) which means that only a small dose (typically 80 MBq) can be given without exposing the patient to unacceptable amounts of radiation. Third, its main emission is the 81 keV mercury X-ray which is of relatively low energy.

These three factors combine to make thallium-201 scintigrams of very low resolution with a low signal to noise ratio. Hence, they are very difficult to interpret without a lot of experience. A further limitation of traditional planar imaging is that the superimposition of normally and abnormally perfused areas reduces the contrast of the abnormal areas and complicates the interpretation of their severity and extent. Fortunately, a number of developments has greatly improved the situation, the most important of which has been the growth of emission tomographic imaging which is to planar imaging as computed X-ray tomography is to the plain chest radiograph.

Advances in myocardial perfusion imaging

Single photon emission computed tomography

In single photon emission computed tomographic imaging, a rotating gamma camera is used to acquire planar images from many projections. This then allows the reconstruction of tomograms in any chosen plane, showing the three-dimensional distribution of thallium-201 throughout the myocardium. The tomograms are much easier to interpret because there is greater contrast between normal and abnormal regions and because cardiologists are more familiar with tomographic anatomy than with projections. Plate 2 shows an example with uniform uptake throughout the myocardium. The clarity of the tomograms compared with conventional planar images is striking. Plate 3 shows an example in a patient with a lesion in the left anterior descending artery before and after coronary angioplasty. The area of reversible ischaemia is relatively small in this patient, hence the patient is at low risk of future events such as myocardial infarction and death. In contrast, Plate 4 shows a 'high-risk' scan with extensive ischaemia and both fixed and reversible defects. Other indicators of high risk are ventricular dilatation in the stress images and high uptake in the lungs. Pulmonary uptake reflects stress-induced elevation of left ventricular end diastolic pressure and transient pulmonary interstitial oedema.

Quantification of images

Computer quantification of the images has helped to make interpretation more objective (Figure 5.1). It is certainly helpful in planar imaging[69,70] but its

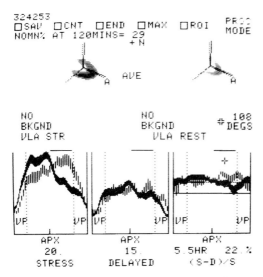

Figure 5.1 Computer quantification of vertical long axis thallium-201 tomograms taken at rest (top right) and during stress (top left). Circumferential profiles are generated by sweeping a radius around the myocardium and the patient profiles (solid lines) are compared with mean profiles from a normal population. The stress profiles (bottom left) show reduced uptake in the anterior wall which normalizes with redistribution (bottom centre). The washout profile (bottom right) shows slow washout from the abnormal area

advantage in tomographic imaging is less clear. Perhaps the reason for this is that the contrast of lesions is so much greater in tomograms that problems of interpretation more frequently involve whether an apparent lesion is due to attenuation or motion of the patient than whether the lesion is present. False-positive defects can be reported in planar images for a variety of reasons, including poor acquisition technique, inexperience, normal variants such as valvar planes and attenuation artefacts, and undue reliance on automated image analysis. In tomographic imaging, the commonest cause of problems is movement of the patient, followed by inadequate quality control of the camera, and attenuation artefacts[71].

Another form of computed analysis is to combine the whole set of short axis tomograms into a single image, called a polar plot or a 'bullseye' display[72,73]. The short axis tomograms are rearranged into concentric circles from apex to base so that all parts of the myocardium are seen in a single display (Figure 5.2). Stress and redistribution images can be generated, each can be compared with known normal ranges, and abnormal areas can be readily identified (Plate 5)[74]. Whilst this is a relatively simple form of analysis, it suffers from being even further from the acquired data than the original tomograms and, hence, susceptible to additional artefacts during reconstruction. It is rare that such polar plots show abnormalities that are not apparent on the tomograms from which they are constructed.

Delayed redistribution

Imaging of myocardial perfusion using thallium-201 traditionally involves the acquisition of images as soon as practical after the injection at peak stress, and again

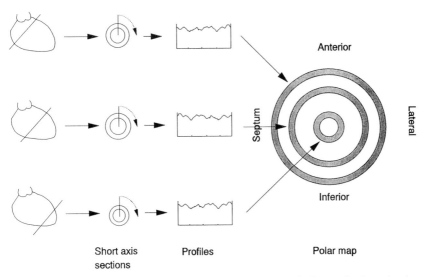

Figure 5.2 Diagrammatic representation of the polar plot, or 'bullseye' display. The short axis tomograms are laid down in a single circular image with the apex in the centre and the base around the periphery

4 h later without further injection. Between the two acquisitions, thallium-201 redistributes into the pattern that it would have had if injected at rest. Defects in both sets of images, therefore, indicate absent or non-viable myocardium. Observation of a defect in the immediate images that normalizes with redistribution indicates an area of viable myocardium that is ischaemic during stress. It has now been demonstrated that redistribution may be incomplete at 4 h in as many as 22% of segments.[75] Even later images may be required if the extent of non-viable myocardium is not to be overestimated. This is not always practical, and an alternative approach if delayed redistribution is suspected is to inject a second dose of thallium-201 at rest. Although this involves an additional burden of radiation, it can be justified in some circumstances. Another method of avoiding 24 hour imaging might be to follow imaging with thallium-201 during stress with imaging using technetium-99m isonitrile at rest, since the 140 keV gamma ray of technetium-99m can be successfully imaged in the presence of thallium-201. Further experimentation is required before an alternative protocol could be recommended for routine use. In the meantime, it is reasonable to continue unchanged, while bearing in mind the possibility of delayed redistribution when planning and reporting studies. The prognostic significance of delayed redistribution appears to be the same as that of early redistribution. It does not necessarily represent more profound ischaemia[76].

Pharmacological stress

A major advantage of imaging of myocardial perfusion is that studies can be performed during pharmacological manipulation of coronary arterial flow as well as during dynamic exercise. This allows reliable information to be obtained in patients who are unable to exercise for non-cardiac reasons such as peripheral vascular disease. The commonest form of pharmacological intervention is dipyridamole[77,78], but adenosine[79] and dobutamine[80] are alternatives. Dipyridamole is a potent coronary arteriolar dilator, and it increases flow approximately five-fold in normal coronary arteries[81]. This contrasts with the 2–3-fold increase caused by maximal dynamic exercise. It acts by inhibiting the enzymatic degradation and cellular uptake of adenosine, which is the direct mediator of vasodilation. Although flow in a normal artery may increase five-fold, the increase in a diseased artery is limited and so differential flow to territories served by normal and stenosed arteries will occur. Such differentials may appear as defects on a thallium-201 image even though the flow in the territory served by the stenosed artery has increased. Dipyridamole can also induce myocardial ischaemia but the mechanisms are poorly understood (Plate 6). One potential mechanism is that the drop in pressure across a stenosis caused by an increase in flow may be so great that the subendocradium is no longer perfused. Another is that an increase in flow in a normal artery which serves a diseased territory by collateral vessels may lead to closure or reversal of flow in the collaterals ('coronary steal').

Myocardial ischaemia occurs in approximately one-third of patients with coronary arterial disease following intravenous dipyridamole[82]. The non-cardiac side-effects are caused by mild peripheral vasodilatation and include flushing, headache, nausea and hypotension. The combination of dynamic exercise with intravenous dipyridamole reduces the incidence of peripheral side-effects and also improves the quality of the images because of splanchnic vasoconstriction[83].

Because of potential myocardial ischaemia, dipyridamole should not be given to patients who would not otherwise be exercised, since there is a small morbidity and mortality, equivalent to that of conventional stress testing[84]. In a recent review of 3911 scans using dipyridamole, four patients (0.1%) suffered myocardial infarction within 24 hours, of whom two died[85]. Three of these patients had unstable angina. Such patients should no longer be considered suitable for infusion of dipyridamole. Ventricular arrhythmias may occur, but they are rarely dangerous. One case of ventricular fibrillation[86] and one of symptomatic bradycardia[87] have been reported. Aminophylline is a specific antagonist and rapidly reverses the action of dipyridamole should adverse reactions occur.

Other radiopharmaceuticals

Although thallium-201 has provided excellent service since its introduction in 1975[88], its physical limitations have led to the search for analogues containing technetium-99m. Two main classes of compound have emerged: the isonitriles[89] and the substituted oximes. A number of early technetium-99m isonitriles suffered from high uptake in the lungs and liver. Methoxyisobutyl isonitrile gives the best imaging of myocardium as compared with background and is now available commercially. Its advantages over thallium-201 are its lower burden of radiation to the patient and the higher resolution of the images that it provides. It is, however, expensive and it has not yet replaced thallium-201 for routine use. Perhaps the most significant difference is that it does not redistribute and so injections are required both at rest and during stress. The two injections can either be given on separate days or, by giving a larger dose for imaging at rest, a same-day protocol is possible. The lack of redistribution brings some advantages in that the injection given during stress need not be given in the nuclear medicine department. Particularly promising studies involve giving the injection immediately before thrombolysis in patients with acute myocardial infarction. Later reinjection and imaging allow the amount of myocardium that has been salvaged by thrombolysis to be established[90].

The second class of technetium-99m myocardial perfusion agents are the boronic adducts of technetium oxime. These have good myocardial uptake with low uptake in the liver and lungs, but they wash out from the myocardium very rapidly so that imaging must be completed within 15–20 minutes of injection. Very rapid imaging may therefore be possible both at rest and during stress.

Positron emission tomography

Although it is not possible to review positron emission tomography in detail, advances in imaging of myocardial perfusion cannot be complete without its mention. Positron emitting radionuclides include carbon-11, nitrogen-13, oxygen-15 and fluorine-18. Their advantage over radionuclides which emit gamma rays is that they are easily incorporated into metabolically active tracers, allowing study of a wide range of pathways in different organs. Their principal disadvantages are their very short half lives (typically seconds or minutes) so that an on-site cyclotron is needed to produce the radionuclides at the point of dispensing, and the requirement for a specialized camera to image their distribution in the body.

In the heart, the main areas of interest for positron emission tomography have been the quantitative assessment of regional myocardial perfusion using rubidium-82 or ^{13}N-ammonia and the imaging of myocardial glucose metabolism using ^{18}F-fluorodexoyglucose. The former allows the non-invasive measurement of the reserve of coronary flow[91] and the latter allows viable but 'hibernating' myocardium to be identified as areas with reduced perfusion in which metabolism has switched from the normal utilization of fatty acids to glucose[92,93]. The significance of this is that it may be possible to identify patients with ischaemic heart failure who do not have angina, but who may benefit from revascularization by the restoration of myocardial function. Because of the expense of positron emission tomography, it is available in only a few research institutions, but cogent arguments have been made that it is a cost-effective method of assessing patients with coronary arterial disease[94].

Conclusion

Myocardial perfusion scintigraphy provides the most accurate method of assessing the site, extent, and severity of the myocardium at risk in patients with coronary arterial disease. Since these factors are very strong determinants of prognosis, the widespread use of the technique should allow a rational method for selecting patients at high risk of future cardiac events, and hence of directing therapeutic measures at those who will benefit most. Recent improvements in techniques of imaging, in particular the development of emission tomographic imaging, have greatly improved their quality. Unfortunately, imaging of myocardial perfusion is still less widely used than it deserves. Appreciation of these developments, and the close involvement of cardiologists in the provision of nuclear cardiological services, should slowly redress the balance so that most patients with coronary arterial disease will then benefit from an objective assessment of the extent of their ischaemia.

References

1. McAfee, J.G., Kopecky, R.T. and Frymoyer, P.A. Nuclear medicine comes of age: its present and future roles in diagnosis. *Radiology*, **174**, 609–20, 1990
2. Kannal, W. and Gordon, T. (eds) *The Framingham Study: An Epidemiological Investigation of Cardiovascular Disease*, DHEW, Washington, DC, publication No. (NIH) 74–599, 1974
3. Wittles, E.H., Hay, J.W. and Gotto, A.M. Medical costs of coronary artery disease in the United States. *Am. J. Cardiol.*, **65**, 432–440, 1990
4. American Heart Association. *Heart Facts*, AKA, Dallas, TX, 1985.
5. European Coronary Surgery Study Group. Prospective randomised study of coronary artery bypass surgery in stable angina pectoris. *Lancet*, **ii**, 491–495, 1980
6. Zir, L.M., Miller, S.W., Dinsmore, R.E., *et al.* Interobserver variability in coronary angiography. *Circulation*, **53**, 627–632, 1976
7. Galbraith, J.E., Murphy, M.L. and Desoyza, N. Coronary angiogram interpretation: interobserver variability. *J. Am. Med. Assoc.*, **240**, 2053–2059, 1981
8. Grodin, C.M., Dyrda, I., Pasternac, A., *et al.* Discrepancies between cine angiographic and post mortem findings in patients with coronary artery disease and recent myocardial revascularisation. *Circulation*, **49**, 703–709, 1974
9. Blankenhorn, D.H. and Curry, P.J. The accuracy of arteriography and ultrasound imaging for atherosclerosis measurement: a review. *Arch. Pathol. Lab. Med.*, **106**, 483–490, 1982
10. Isner, J.M., Kishel, J. and Kent, K.M. Accuracy of angiographic determination of left main coronary arterial narrowing. *Circulation*, **63**, 1056–1061, 1981
11. Roberts, W.C. and Jones, A.A. Quantitation of coronary arterial narrowing at necropsy in sudden coronary death. *Am. J. Cardiol.*, **44**, 38–44, 1979
12. Vlodaver, Z., Frech, R., van Tassel, R.A. and Edwards, J.E. Correlation of the antemortem coronary angiogram and the postmortem specimen. *Circulation*, **47**, 162–168, 1973
13. White, C.W., Wright, C.B., Doty, D.B., *et al.* Does visual interpretation of the coronary arteriogram predict the physiologic importance of a coronary stenosis? *N. Engl. J. Med.*, **310**, 819–824, 1984
14. Balcon, R. Prognostic significance of coronary angiography. *Eur. Heart J.*, **5**, 73–75, 1984
15. Balcon, R. The relationship between prognosis and angiographic and exercise data. *Acta Med. Scand.*, **694** (suppl), 101–103, 1984
16. Moise, A., Clement, B. and Saltiel, J. Clinical and angiographic correlates and prognostic significance of the coronary extent score. *Am. J. Cardiol.*, **61**, 1255–1259, 1988
17. Nissen, S.E. and Gurley, J.C. Assessment of the functional significance of coronary stenoses. Is digital angiography the answer? *Circulation*, **81**, 1431–1435, 1990
18. Chesebro, J.H., Fuster, V. and Webster, M.W.I. Editorial comment. Endothelial injury and coronary vasomotion. *J. Am. Coll. Cardiol.*, **14**, 1191–1192, 1989
19. Bing, R.J. Editorial comment. Control of shear stress in the epicardial coronary arteries of humans: impairment by atherosclerosis. *J. Am. Coll. Cardiol.*, **14**, 1200–1201, 1989
20. Vita, J.A., Treasure, C.B., Ganz, P., *et al.* Control of shear stress in the epicardial coronary arteries of humans: impairment by atherosclerosis. *J. Am. Coll. Cardiol.*, **14**, 1193–1199, 1989
21. Chaitman, B.R. The changing role of the exercise electrocardiogram as a diagnostic and prognostic test for chronic ischemic heart disease. *J. Am. Coll. Cardiol.*, **8**, 1195–1210, 1986
22. Rautaharju, P.M., Prineas, R.J., Eifler, W.J., *et al.* Prognostic value of exercise electrocardiogram in men at high risk of future coronary heart disease: multiple risk factor intervention trial experience. *J. Am. Coll. Cardiol.*, **8**, 1–10, 1986
23. Stone, P.H., Turi, Z.G., Muller, J.E., *et al.* Prognostic significance of the treadmill exercise test performance 6 months after myocardial infarction. *J. Am. Coll. Cardiol.*, **8**, 1007–1017, 1986
24. Goldschlager, N. and Sox, H.C. The diagnostic and prognostic value of the treadmill exercise test in the evaluation of chest pain, in patients with recent myocardial infarction, and in asymptomatic individuals. *Am. Heart J.*, **116**, 523–535, 1988
25. Elamin, M.S., Boyle, R., Kardash, M.M., *et al.* Accurate detection of coronary heart disease by new exercise test. *Br. Heart J.*, **48**, 311–320, 1982
26. Fox, K.M. Exercise heart rate/ST segment relation. Perfect predictor of coronary disease? *Br. Heart J.*, **48**, 309–310, 1982
27. Finkelhor, R.S., Newhouse, K.E., Vrobel, T.R., *et al.* The ST segment/heart rate slope as a predictor of coronary artery disease: comparison with quantitative thallium imaging and conventional ST segment criteria. *Am. Heart J.*, **112**, 296–304, 1986
28. Borer, J.S., Bacharach, S.L., Green, M.V., *et al.* Real-time radionuclide cineangiography in the noninvsaive evaluation of global and regional left ventricular function at rest and during exercise in patients with coronary artery disease. *N. Engl. J. Med.*, **296**, 839–844, 1977

29. Borer, J.S., Kent, K.M., Bacharach, S.L., *et al.* Sensitivity, specificity and predictive accuracy of radionuclide cineangiography during exercise in patients with coronary artery disease. Comparison with exercise eleccardiography. *Circulation*, **60**, 572–580, 1979
30. Bodenheimer, M.M., Banka, V.S., Fooshee, C.M. and Helfant, R.H. Comparative sensitivity of the exercise electrocardiogram, thallium imaging and stress radionuclide angiography to detect the presence and severity of coronary heart disease. *Circulation*, **60**, 1270–1278, 1979
31. Berger, H.J., Reduto, L.A., Johnstone, D.E., *et al.* Global and regional left ventricular response to bicycle exercise artery disease. Assessment by quantitative radionuclide angiocardiography. *Am. J. Med.*, **66**, 13–21, 1979
32. Becker, L.C. Diagnosis of coronary artery disease with exercise radionuclide imaging: state of the art. *Am. J. Cardiol.*, **45**, 1301–1304, 1980
33. Austin, E.H., Cobb, F.R., Coleman, R.E. and Jones, R.H. Prospective evaluation of radionuclide angiocardiography for the diagnosis of coronary artery disease. *Am. J. Cardiol.*, **50**, 1212–1216, 1982
34. O'Keefe, J.C., Cooper, R.A., Edwards, A.C., *et al.* Comparison of exercise electrocardiography, thallium-201 myocardial imaging and exercise gated blood pool scan in patients with suspected coronary artery disease. *Austr. N. Z. J. Med.*, **13**, 45–50, 1983
35. Rozanski, A., Diamond, G., Berman, D., *et al.* The declining specificity of exercise radionuclide ventriculography. *N. Engl. J. Med.*, **309**, 518–522, 1983
36. Beller, G.A. Nuclear Cardiology: current indications and clinical usefulness. *Curr. Prob. Cardiol.*, **10**, 3–76, 1985
37. Marcus, M.L., White, C.W. and Kirchner, P.T. Isn't it time to reevaluate the sensitivity of noninvasive approaches for the diagnosis of coronary artery disease? *J. Am. Coll. Cardiol.*, **8**, 1033–1034, 1986
38. Underwood, S.R., Walton, S., Laming, P.J., *et al.* Quantitative phase analysis in the assessment of coronary artery disease. *Br. Heart J.*, **61**, 14–22, 1989
39. Plotnick, G.D. and Vogel, R.A. Noninvasive evaluation of diastolic function: need for hemodynamically and clinically relevant variables. *J. Am. Coll. Cardiol.*, **13**, 1015–1016, 1989
40. Dewhurst, N.G. and Muir, A.L. Comparative prognostic value of radionuclide ventriculography at rest and during exercise in 100 parients after first myocardial infarction. *Br. Heart R.*, **49**, 111–121, 1983.
41. Pryor, D.B., Harrell, F.E. Jr, Lee K.L., *et al.* Prognostic indicators from radionuclide angiography in medically treated parients with coronary artery disease. *Am. J. Cardiol.*, **53**, 18–22, 1984
42. Bonow, R.O., Kent, K.M., Rosing, D.R., *et al.* Exercise-induced ischaemia in mildly symptomatic patients with coronary artery disease, and preserved left ventricular function: identification of subgroups at high risk for death during medical therapy. *N. Engl. J. Med.*, **311**, 1339–1345, 1984
43. Fioretti, P., Brower, R.W., Simoons, M.L., *et al.* Prediction of mortality in hospital survivors of myocardial infarction. Comparison of predischarge exercise testing and radionuclide ventriculography at rest. *Br. Heart J.*, **52**, 292–298, 1984
44. Iskandrian, A.S., Hakki, A.H., Goel, I.P., *et al.* The use of rest and exercise radionuclide ventriculography in risk stratification in patients with suspected coronary artery disease. *Am. Heart J.*, **110**, 864–872, 1985
45. Gillespie, J.A. and Moss, A.J. Postinfarction risk profiling: past, present and future considerations. *J. Am. Coll. Cardiol.*, **8**, 50–51, 1986
46. Corne, R.A. Risk stratification in stable angina pectoris. *Am. J. Cardiol.*, **59**, 695–697, 1987
47. Abraham, R.D., Harris, P.J., Roubin, G.S., *et al.* Usefulness of ejection fraction response to exercise one month after acute myocardial infarction in predicting coronary anatomy and prognosis. *Am. J. Cardiol.*, **60**, 225–230, 1987
48. Brown, K.A., Boucher, C.A., Okada, R.D., *et al.* Prognostic value of exercise thallium-201 imaging in patients presenting for evaluation of chest pain. *J. Am. Coll. Cardiol.*, **1**, 994–1001, 1983
49. Koss, J.H., Kobren, S.M., Grunwald, A.M. and Bodenheimer, M.M. Role of exercise thallium-201 myocardial perfusion scintigraphy in predicting prognosis in suspected coronary artery disease. *Am. J. Cardiol.*, **59**, 531–534, 1987
50. Iskandrian, A.S., Heo, J., Decoskey, D., *et al.* Use of exercise thallium-201 imaging for risk stratification of elderly patients with coronary artery dissease. *Am. J. Cardiol.*, **61**, 269–272, 1988
51. Kaul, S., Finkelstein, D.M., Homma, S., *et al.* Superiority of quantitative exercise thallium-201 variables in determining long-term prognosis in ambulatory patients with chest pain: a comparison with cardiac catheterization. *J. Am. Coll. Cardiol.*, **12**, 25–34, 1988
52. Bairey, C.N., Rozanski, A., Maddahi, J., *et al.* Exercise thallium-201 scintigraphy and prognosis in typical angina pectoris and negative exercixe electrocardiography. *Am. J. Cardiol.*, **64**, 282–287, 1989

53. Hendel, R.C., Layden, J.J. and Leppo, J.A. Prognostic value of dipyridamole thallium scintigraphy for evaluation of ischemic heart disease. *J. Am. Coll. Cardiol.*, **15**, 109–16, 1990

54. Gibson, R.S., Watson, D.D., Craddock, G.B., *et al.* Prediction of cardiac events after uncomplicated myocardial infarction: a prospective study comparing predischarge exercise thallium-201 scintigraphy and coronary angiography. *Circulation*, **68**, 321–336, 1983

55. Leppo, J.A., O'Brien, J., Rothendler, J.A., *et al.* Dipyridamole-thallium-201 scintigraphy in the prediction of future cardiac events after acute myocardial infarction. *N. Engl. J. Med.*, **310**, 1014–1018, 1984

56. Wilson, W.W., Gibson, R.S., Nygaard, T.W., *et al.* Acute myocardial infarction associated with single vessel coronary artery disease: an analysis of clinical outcome and the prognostic importance of vessel patency and residual ischemic myocardium. *J. Am. Coll. Cardiol.*, **11**, 223–234, 1988

57. Gimple, L.W., Hutter, A.M., Guiney, T.E. and Boucher, C.A. Prognostic utility of predischarge dipyridamole-thallium imaging compared to predischarge submaximal exercise electrocardiography and maximal exercise thallium imaging after uncomplicated acute myocardial infarction. *Am. J. Cardiol.*, **64**, 1243–1248, 1989

58. Younis, L.T., Byers, S., Shaw, L. *et al.* Prognostic value of intravenous dipyridamole thallium scintigraphy after an acute myocardial ischemic event. *Am. J. Cardiol.*, **64**, 161–166, 1989

59. Younis, L.T., Byers, S., Shaw, L., *et al.* Prognostic importance of silent myocardial ischaemia detected by intravenous dipyridamole thallium myocardial perfusion imaging in asymptomatic patients with coronary artery disease. *J. Am. Coll. Cardiol.*, **14**, 1635–1641, 1990

60. Fleg, J.L., Gerstenblith, G., Zonderman, A.B., *et al.* Prevalence and prognostic significance of exercise-induced silent myocardial ischaemia detected by thallium scintigraphy and electrocardiography in asymptomatic volunteers. *Circulation*, **81**, 428–436, 1990

61. Ladenheim, M.L., Pollock, B.H., Rozanski, A., *et al.* Extent and severity of myocardial perfusion as predictors of prognosis in patients with suspected coronary artery disease. *J. Am. Coll. Cardiol.*, **3**, 464–471, 1986

62. Ladenheim, M.L., Kotler, T.S., Pollock, B.H., *et al.* Incremental prognostic power of clinical history, exercise electrocardiography and myocardial perfusion scintigraphy in suspected coronary artery disease. *Am. J. Cardiol.*, **59**, 270–277, 1987

63. Anderson, H.V., Talley, J.D., Black, A.J.R., *et al.* Usefulness of coronary angioplasty in asymptomatic patients. *Am. J. Cardiol.*, **65**, 35–39, 1990

64. Little, W.C., Constantinescu, M., Applegate, R.J., *et al.* Can coronary angiography predict the site of a subsequent myocardial infarction in patients with mild-to-moderate coronary artery disease? *Circulation*, **78**, 1157–1166, 1988

65. Hackett, D., Davies, G. and Maseri, A. Pre-existing coronary stenoses in patients with first myocardial infarction are not necessarily severe. *Eur. Heart J.*, **9**, 1317–1323, 1988

66. Brosius, F.C. and Roberts, W.C. Comparison of degree and extent of coronary narrowing by atherosclerotic plaque in anterior and posterior transmural acute myocardial infarction. *Circulation*, **64**, 715–722, 1981

67. Underwood, S.R., Gibson, C.J., Tweddel, A. and Flint, J. Survey of nuclear cardiology practice in Great Britain in 1988. *Nucl. Med. Commun.*, **10**, 258–259 (Abstract), 1989

68. Subcommittee of the Health and Environment Research Advisory Committee, Office of Energy Research, US Department of Energy. *Review of the Office of Health and Environment Research Program, Nuclear Medicine, 1989*, US Department of Energy, Washington, DC, 1989

69. Beller, G.A. Quantitative thallium-201 scintigraphy. *Int. J. Cardiol.*, **5**, 234–239, 1984

70. Reisman, S., Maddahi, J., Van Train, K., *et al.* Quantitation of extent, depth and severity of planar thallium defects in patients undergoing exercise thallium-201 scintigraphy. *J. Nucl. Med.*, **27**, 1273–1281, 1986

71. DePuey, E.G. and Garcia, E.V. Optimal specificity of thallium-201 SPECT through recognition of imaging artifacts. *J. Nucl. Med.*, **30**, 441–449, 1989

72. Garcia, E.V., Van Train, K., Maddahi, J., *et al.* Quantitation of rotational thallium-201 myocardial perfusion tomography. *J. Nucl. Med.*, **26**, 17–26, 1985

73. DePasquale, E.E., Nody, A.C., DePuey, E.G., *et al.* Quantative rotational thallium-201 tomography for identifying and localising coronary artery disease. *Circulation*, **77**, 316–327, 1988

74. Mahmarian, J.J., Boyce, T.M., Goldberg, R.K., *et al.* Quantitative exercise thallium-201 single photon emission computed tomography for the enhanced diagnosis of ischaemic heart disease. *J. Am. Coll. Cardiol.*, **15**, 318–329, 1990

75. Yang, L.D., Berman, D.S., Kiat, H., *et al.* The frequency of late reversibility in SPECT thallium-201 stress-redistribution studies. *J. Am. Coll. Cardiol.*, **15**, 334–340, 1990

76. Botvinick, E.H. Late reversibility: a viability issue. *J. Am. Coll. Cardiol.*, **15**, 341–344, 1990

77. Leppo, J., Boucher, C.A., Okada, R.D., *et al*. Serial thallium-201 myocardial imaging after dipyridamole infusion: diagnostic utility in detecting coronary stenoses and relationship to regional wall motion. *Circulation*, **66**, 649–657, 1982

78. Iskandrian, A.S., Heo, J., Askenase, A., *et al*. Dipyridamole cardiac imaging. *Am. Heart J.*, **115**, 432–43, 1988

79. Siffring, P.A., Gupta, N.C., Mohiuddin, S.M., *et al*. Myocardial uptake and clearance of T1-201 in healthy subjects: comparison of adenosine-induced hyperemia and exercise stress. *Radiology*, **173**, 769–774, 1989

80. *Lancet*. Dobutamine stress test. *Lancet*, **ii**, 1347–1348, 1988

81. Gould, K.L., Noninvasive assessment of coronary stenoses by myocardial perfusion imaging during pharmacologic coronary vasodilation. I. Physiologic basis and experimental validation. *Am. J. Cardiol.*, **41**, 267–278, 1978

82. Pennell, D.J., Underwood, S.R., Ell, P.J., *et al*. Magnetic resonance imaging using dipyridamole: a comparison with thallium-201 emission tomography. *Br. Heart J.*, **64**, 362–369, 1990

83. Walker, P.R., James, M.A., Wilde, R.P.H., *et al*. Dipyridamole combined with exercise for thallium myocardial imaging. *Br. Heart J.*, **55**, 321–329, 1986

84. Gibbons, L., Blair, S.N., Kohl, H.W. and Cooper, K. The safety of maximal exercise testing. *Circulation*, **80**, 846–852, 1989

85. Ranhosky, A. and Kempthorne-Rawson, J. The safety of intravenous dipyridamole thallium myocardial perfusion imaging. *Circulation*, **81**, 1205–1209, 1990

86. Bayliss, J., Pearson, M. and Sutton, G.C. Ventricular dysrhythmias following intravenous dipyridamole during stress myocardial imaging. *Br. J. Radiol.*, **56**, 686, 1983

87. Pennell, D.J., Underwood, S.R. and Ell, P.J. Symptomatic bradycardia complicating the use of intravenous dipyridamole for thallium-201 myocardial perfusion imaging. *Int. J. Cardiol.*, **27**, 272–274, 1990

88. Lebowitz, E., Green, M.W., Fairchild, R., *et al*. Thallium-201 for medical use. *J. Nucl. Med.*, **16**, 151–155, 1975

89. Jones, A.G., Abrams, M.J. and Davison, A. A new class of water soluble low valent technetium unipositive cations: hexakisisontrile technetium(I) salts. *J. Nucl. Med. Allied Sci.*, **26**, 149, 1982

90. Wackers, F.J.T., Gibbons, R.J., Verani, M.S., *et al*. Serial quantitative planar technetium-99m isonitrile imaging in acute myocardial infarction: efficacy for noninvasive assessment of thrombolytic therapy. *J. Am. Coll. Cardiol.*, **14**, 861–873, 1989

91. Gould, K.L., Goldstein, R.A., Mullani, N.A., *et al*. Noninvasive assessment of coronary stenosis by myocardial perfusion imaging during pharmacologic coronary vasodilation. VIII. Clinical feasibility of positron cardiac imaging without a cyclotron using a generator-produced rubidium-82. *J. Am. Coll. Cardiol.*, **7**, 775–789, 1986

92. Brunken, R., Tillisch, J., Schwaiger, M., *et al*. Regional perfusion, glucose metabolism and wall motion in chronic electrocardiographic Q-wave infarctions: evidence for persistence of viable tissue in some infarct regions by positron emission tomography. *Circulation*, **73**, 951–963, 1986

93. Tillisch, J., Brunken, R., Marshall, R., *et al*. Reversibility of cardiac wall motion abnormalities predicted by using positron tomography. *N. Engl. J. Med.*, **314**, 884–888, 1986

94. Gould, K.L., Goldstein, R.A. and Mullani, N.A. Economic analysis of clinical positron emission tomography of the heart with rubidium-82. *J. Nucl. Med.*, **30**, 707–717, 1989

6

A macroscopic and microscopic view of the insult to the coronary arteries in ischaemic heart disease

Jessica M. Mann and Michael J. Davies

Introduction

Coronary arterial disease can be either fixed or dynamic, depending on the morphology of the atherosclerotic plaque. Concentric plaques will affect the entire circumference of the media, whereas eccentric plaques keep an area of normal medial muscle, thus allowing changes in the diameter of the lumen.

Coronary arterial thrombosis, in contrast, depends on the presence of intimal injury, which can be just an extension of the endothelial denudation seen in intact plaques, or a fissure in the plaque leading to a deeper injury. In the latter, fissures extend to the lipid pool. Thus the thrombus starts within the plaque. This thrombus can later increase in size, becoming mural or occlusive, or be 'reabsorbed' into the plaque, leading to an increase in total plaque area. Unstable plaques (those with fissures) are most commonly found in patients with unstable angina, acute myocardial infarction and sudden cardiac death. Contributory factors to fissuring of the plaque are a high local tensile stress and infiltration of the matrix of connective tissue by macrophages. It is these various features of the pathology of coronary arterial disease that are discussed in this review.

The atherosclerotic plaque

The atherosclerotic plaque is the typical lesion of atherosclerosis. These plaques can be seen on the arterial intima as raised yellow deposits, and they may be covered by fibrous tissue. The best way of assessing the degree of arterial stenosis produced by such plaques is by evaluating transverse cuts of the affected arteries. Prior perfusion at arterial pressures, however, should always be performed so as to keep the arterial lumen circular. Atherosclerotic plaques consist mainly of lipids and collagen (Figure 6.1). The earliest atherosclerotic lesion, seen in infants [1], consists of accumulation of lipids within macrophages. These cholesterol esters derive from cholesterol present within the plasma [2]. Fatty streaks show intra- and extracellular accumulation of such esters, while the content of extracellular lipids is even higher in the typical atherosclerotic plaque. Most of these plaques have a large core of amorphous lipid which contains crystals of cholesterol [2]. Techniques using monoclonal antibodies have been used to identify those cells with deposits of lipids, as well as the cells forming the fibrous cap around the lipid core. The former were shown to be macrophages, and the latter smooth muscle cells [3]. These smooth muscle cells are

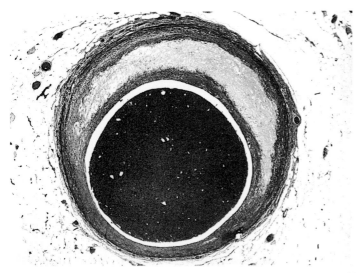

Figure 6.1 Transverse section of a coronary artery showing the crescent-like lipid pool surrounded by a fibrous cap. The lumen of the artery is filled with contrast medium

also responsible for the synthesis of collagen, which in atherosclerotic plaques is mostly of types I and III.

Atherosclerotic plaques within the coronary arteries can be classified as concentric or eccentric. These morphological differences have major functional significance. Necropsy studies [4] have shown that, in transverse sections of coronary arteries with more than a 75% decrease in the cross-sectional area, the thickness of the media is substantially reduced, either due to atrophy of the smooth muscle or to 'invasion' by the atherosclerotic plaque. The extent of medial thinning – or atrophy – depends mainly on the morphology of the plaque. Concentric lesions generally show even greater involvement of the media, whereas eccentric lesions maintain an area of normal medial muscle. This area of normal medial muscle is thought to be responsible for a 'variable' degree of coronary arterial narrowing [5], since the muscle that is normal would be able to respond to different stimuli, such as those triggering spasm. This dynamic process is not seen in concentric lesions, since no normal muscle is retained to respond to the same stimuli.

Necropsy studies of patients with stable angina have shown that 76% of the atherosclerotic lesions within the coronary arteries were concentric and, of these, most were fibrous (48%) [6]. Other studies [7], however, have shown a predominance of eccentric high-grade lesions. Patients with stable angina will clearly have at least one high-grade eccentric lesion, with a variable cross-sectional area, which can be held, at least partially, responsible for any acute events [6].

High-grade stenosis (greater than 50% reduction in diameter) have been shown to have a higher proportion of fibrous tissue than stenosis of less than 50% [6], probably because the fibrous tissue has replaced a lipid pool which underwent early thrombosis and, later, organization. Furthermore, most (79%) of the patients with stable angina have been shown, at necropsy, to have a multichannelled arterial lumen, implying recanalization of a previous thrombus some time in their cardiological history.

The lipid pool seen in the atherosclerotic plaques also shows great variation. It can be generally seen as a crescent, surrounded by a fibrous cap which isolates it from the arterial lumen (Figure 6.1). Most of these lipids are extracellular, mainly cholesterol esters similar to esters of low density lipoproteins. The size of the lipid pool, as well as that of the fibrous cap, shows a huge individual variation. Monocytes and T lymphocytes [3] are present around the lipid pool, once again in variable amounts. It remains to be determined whether different plaques represent different steps in the same evolving process or are truly different lesions. Most of the patients with atherosclerotic coronary arterial disease have a population of plaques of mixed morphology.

The endothelium

The normal endothelium consists of a single layer of cells with several important functions defined recently, such as the production of growth factors [8] and vasoactive agents. This endothelial layer remains intact in fatty streaks, but not in raised plaques. Removal of the endothelium leads to exposure of collagen, which then attracts platelets. This process is initiated mainly by the interaction of the glycoproteins Ia and Ib contained in the membranes of platelets within the subendothelium. Since the endothelial layer is intact in fatty streaks, there is no possible interaction with platelets and the subendothelium. This fact, therefore, cannot be considered the main triggering event for the appearance of the plaque. On the other hand, once endothelial injury is present, it may be a stimulus for proliferation of smooth muscle, probably through release of growth factors [8]. The only method for assessment of endothelial injury or denudation is perfusion of the vessel immediately after death, although explanted hearts of patients undergoing heart transplantation offer an alternative model [9].

Thrombosis and atherosclerotic plaques

Whenever the endothelial layer is discontinuous, platelets adhere to the subendothelium by a complex interaction between their glycoprotein receptors and the exposed subendothelial collagen [10]. Once the layer of adhesive platelets is established, platelet aggregation is started by different pathways (arachidonate, adenosine diphosphate or collagen–thrombin) [10]. Fibrinogen and fibronectin activate more platelets and the clotting mechanism can be activated by contact between blood and the subendothelium. As soon as thrombin is produced, it triggers formation of fibrin, which leads to stabilization of the platelets and adherence of the thrombus to the arterial wall. The rate of growth of the thrombus depends on flow and on the depth of the intimal injury. The deeper the injury, the higher the likelihood of thrombosis.

Necropsy studies (Davies, unpublished observations) have shown that most (74.7%) of thrombi occur on plaques with intimal fissures and tears. Whenever thrombi were unassociated with tears of plaques, there was endothelial denudation and a severe underlying stenosis. Of thrombi lying on an intact plaque, 81% had an underlying stenosis greater than 60% by diameter. Reduction in diameter produced by the plaque alone was below 30% in 13% of cases, 40% in 13%, 50% in 16%, 60% in 20%, 70% in 15% and greater than 80% in 15%. The relationship between non-severe stenosis, plaque fissuring and lethal thrombosis has also been corroborated angiographically in patients with acute myocardial infarction [11]. The difference between a superficial thrombus on an intact plaque and a deep thrombus on a fissured plaque was recognized more than 15 years ago [12]. Deep intimal tears have a more extensive surface of collagen interacting with platelets, thus producing bigger thrombi, and the thrombus starts within the plaque. The location of the thrombus within the plaques leads to an increase in area and further reduction of the arterial lumen and flow of blood, which could result in further formation of thrombus. Also, whenever there is an area of normal medial muscle, the possibility of arterial spasm due to tearing of the plaque and deposition of platelets has to be considered.

Intimal tears range in size from fissures (quantitated in μm) to cracks (of size measured in mm) to rupture (loss of the whole cap). Such variability in lesions was already described in 1926 [13]. Later, angiographic studies during necropsies [14] showed that 78.9% of coronary arterial stenosis were of so-called type II (that is, eccentric lesions with an irregular or scalloped border) while intraluminal filling defects were shown histologically to be 'complicated' lesions (showing plaque rupture, haemorrhage, occlusive thrombus or recanalized thrombus). Subsequently, angiographic studies in patients with acute myocardial infarction [11], unstable angina [15] and in some patients resuscitated from sudden death showed the same appearances in the nature of the coronary stenosis (that is, so-called type II lesions).

Thrombosis related to fissuring of a plaque has three stages, all of them identified through necropsy studies performed in patients dying from coronary disease. In the first, or early, stage the intima is torn, allowing the lipids within the plaque to interact with the arterial blood. The result is formation of a thrombus within the intima, but none within the arterial lumen. This intimal thrombus is composed mainly of platelets. The second, or intermediate, stage consists of extension of the same intimal thrombus into the arterial lumen through the fissure in the plaque. This 'luminal' component is mural, thus allowing antegrade blood flow. This second stage in thrombosis corresponds with the production of mural thrombi seen in patients with unstable angina and acute myocardial infarction (so-called type II stenosis) [16]. The third, or final, stage is the occlusion of the arterial lumen by expansion of the thrombus. Occlusive thrombi have a much greater proportion of fibrin than do non-occlusive thrombi, and this mesh of fibrin extends distally into the arterial lumen, thus occluding it. Non-occlusive thrombi are responsible for generating the small platelet thrombi which embolize in the territory of the artery containing the fissured plaque [7,8]. Crystals of cholesterol coming from the ulcerated plaque can also embolize into the distal vessel.

Thrombi in this third or last stage are susceptible to fibrinolysis, whether endogenous or exogenous. Studies of patients receiving thrombolytic therapy in the early stages of acute myocardial infarction [19] showed intermittent reopening and reocclusion of the arteries affected. Coronary angiograms during fibrinolysis show a rapid restoration of antegrade blood flow around the silhouette of the intraluminal thrombus. This thrombus decreases in size with time elapsed, but generally the mural component, richer in fibrin, remains adherent to the arterial wall [20]. The underlying fissured plaque can be seen as an irregular (or type II) stenosis. Necropsy studies of patients dying after fibrinolysis are scarce [21], but the few available show that, when the intraluminal thrombus is lysed, the underlying fissured plaque can be seen. The fate of the intraintimal thrombus, however, is still under discussion. Necropsy studies of successful versus unsuccessful thrombolysis [22] show that complex plaque fissures are most frequent when thrombolysis has been unsuccessful. Whenever the fissure is very large, a flap of intima can be raised with extrusion of cholesterol·and collagen into the lumen. Or, if most of the thrombus lies within the intima, the lumen will be compressed. Fibrinolysis will not be helpful in these situations.

The role of cholesterol within the arterial lumen in relation to the outcome of fibrinolysis remains to be determined. Intraluminal thrombi contain crystals of cholesterol, which probably end up in the distal arterial bed after fibrinolysis. The final effect of these crystals on coronary flow reserve is unknown. Percutaneous transluminal coronary angioplasty combined with fibrinolytic therapy can produce compression of the arterial lumen due to haemorrhage within both the intima and the media [21]. On the other hand, angioplasty by itself produces deeper tears in the plaque, sometimes reaching the adventitia, thereby increasing the risk of formation of haematoma.

Plaque fissures

Plaque fissures can be found in coronary arteries of patients dying of non-cardiac diseases and used as controls in necropsy studies. Their frequency is 8.7% in non-hypertensive, non-diabetic patients [23] and this increases to 16.7% in patients with hypertension or diabetes. Intraluminal thrombi, however, are very rare in these control hearts. Patients suffering sudden death, acute myocardial infarction or unstable angina have a much higher incidence of fissured plaques and of intraluminal thrombi [24,25]. The immediate consequence of fissuring is an increase in the volume of the plaque, due first to the thrombus inside the plaque and, later, to growth of collagen when the thrombus becomes organized. Sequential coronary angiographic studies have demonstrated the progression of lesions leading eventually to severe stenosis [26], the underlying mechanism being formation of a fissure. The formation of intraluminal thrombi is also stimulated by plaque fissuring and, although individual

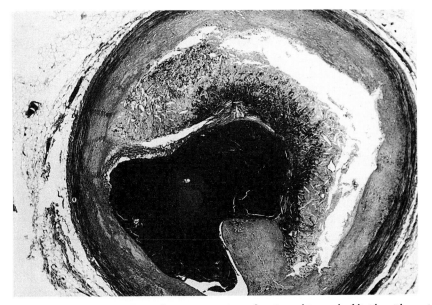

Figure 6.2 Transverse section of a coronary artery showing a big pool of lipids with crystals of cholesterol. There is a fissure of the fibrous cap and an intraluminal occlusive thrombus

balance between thrombolysis and thrombogenesis may be the most important factor, the size of the fissure remains one of its main determinants.

Spontaneously occurring intimal tears can be compared with the intimal injuries seen after coronary angioplasty, since the healing processes are very similar. If the fissure is small, proliferation of smooth muscle will seal it up and keep the thrombus within the plaque. When the thrombus becomes organized, the plaque will be invaded by vessels and fibroblasts from the media leading to an increase in the area of the plaque. Hence, plaque fissuring and thrombosis (Figure 6.2) can result in an increase in area of the plaque, in residual severe stenosis (either with a single-channel lumen or a multichannelled lumen), or in occlusion (Figure 6.3).

Intraluminal thrombi appear when there is a fissure connecting the arterial lumen with the plaque (Figure 6.2). Most of the intraluminal thrombus is formed by platelets, which, in turn, aggregate further platelets within the intima by release of adenosine diphosphate and other factors. Whenever the fibrous cap surrounding the

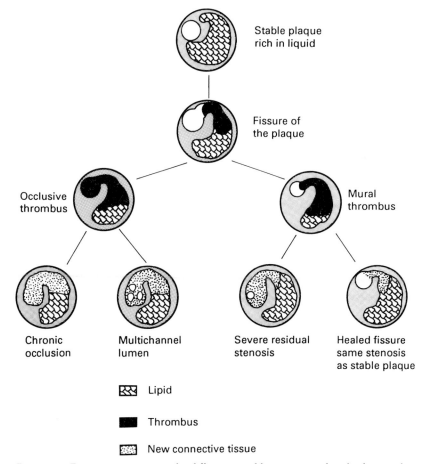

Figure 6.3 Diagram representing the different possible outcomes after the fissure of an atherosclerotic plaque. These can go from a chronic total occlusion to healing of the fissure, the latter resulting in no increase in the pre-existing degree of coronary arterial stenosis

lipid pool is intact, no platelets are seen on the plaque, although some erythrocytes may be present. These erythrocytes may come from vessels newly formed in the media. Step sectioning of the arteries is a useful technique to demonstrate the fissure which allows platelets to enter the intima and form an intraintimal haematoma.

Mechanism of plaque fissuring

Necropsy studies of fissured and thrombosed plaques have shown that, in 83% of them, the tear extended into a pool of extracellular lipid with no buttressing by collagen from beneath [27]. The weak spot on the plaque was generally the site where the fibrous cap was attached to a relatively normal vessel wall. Computer models of atherosclerotic vessel walls have shown that plaques with a deformable core of lipid have a high systolic stress at the junction of normal and abnormal arterial wall. When there is a very rigid material present such as calcium, the shear stress induced locally rises, leading to intimal tears in calcified plaques.

References

1. Stary, H.C. Evolution and progression of atherosclerotic lesions in coronary arteries of children and young adults. *Arteriosclerosis*, **9** (Suppl. 1), 19–32, 1989
2. Lundberg, B. Chemical composition and physical state of lipid deposits in atherosclerosis. *Atherosclerosis*, **56**, 93–110, 1985
3. Johasson, L., Holm, J., Skalli, O., *et al.* Regional accumulations of T cells, macrophages, and smooth muscle cells in the human atherosclerotic plaque. *Arteriosclerosis*, **6**, 131–138, 1986
4. Isner, J.M., Donaldson, R.F., Fortin, A.H., *et al.* Attenuation of the media of coronary arteries in advanced atherosclerosis. *Am. J. Cardiol.*, **58**, 937–939, 1986
5. Saner, H.E., Gobel, F.L., Salomonowitz, E., *et al.* The disease-free wall in coronary atherosclerosis: its relation to degree of obstruction. *J. Am. Coll. Cardiol.*, **6**, 1096–1099, 1985
6. Hangartner, J.R.W., Charleston, A.J., Davies, M.J. and Thomas, A.C. Morphological characteristics of clinically significant coronary artery stenosis in stable angina. *Br. Heart J.*, **56**, 501–508, 1986
7. Freudenberg, H. and Lichtlen, P. Das normale Wandsegment bei Koronarstenosen, eine postmortale Studie. *Z. Kardiol.*, **70**, 863–869, 1981
8. Ross, R. The pathogenesis of atherosclerosis – an update. *N. Engl. J. Med.*, **314**, 488–500, 1986
9. Davies, M.J., Woolf, N., Rowles, P.M. and Pepper, J. Morphology of the endothelium over atherosclerotic plaques in human coronary arteries. *Br. Heart J.*, **60**, 459–464, 1988
10. Fuster, V., Badimon, L., Cohen, M., *et al.* Insights into the pathogenesis of acute ischemic syndromes. *Circulation*, **77**, 1213–1220, 1988
11. Ambrose, J.A., Tannenbaum, M.A., Alexopoulos, D., *et al.* Angiographic progression of coronary artery disease and the development of myocardial infarction. *J. Am. Coll. Cardiol.*, **12**, 56–62, 1988
12. Chandler, A.B. Mechanisms and frequency of thrombosis in the coronary circulation. *Thromb. Res.*, **4**, 3–23, 1974
13. Benson, R.L. The present status of coronary arterial disease. *Arch. Pathol.*, **2**, 876–916, 1926
14. Levin, D.C. and Fallon, J.T. Significance of the angiographic morphology of localised coronary stenoses: histopathologic correlations. *Circulation*, **66**, 316–320, 1982
15. Ambrose, J.A., Winters, S.L., Arora, R.R., *et al.* Angiographic evolution of coronary artery morphology in unstable angina. *J. Am. Coll. Cardiol.*, **7**, 472–478, 1986
16. Ambrose, J.A., Winters, S.L., Arora, R., *et al.* Coronary angiographic morphology in myocardial infarction: a link between the pathogenesis of unstable angina and myocardial infarction. *J. Am. Coll. Cardiol.*, **6**, 1233–1238, 1985
17. Frink, R.J., Rooney, P.A., Trowbridge, J.O. and Rose, J.P. Coronary thrombosis and platelet/fibrin microemboli in death associated with acute myocardial infarction. *Br. Heart J.*, **59**, 196–200, 1988
18. Davies, M.J., Thomas, A.C., Knapman, P.A. and Hangartner, J.R. Intramyocardial platelet aggregation in patients with unstable angina suffering sudden ischemic cardiac death. *Circulation*, **73**, 418–427, 1986

19. Hackett, D., Davies, G., Chierchia, S. and Maseri, A. Intermittent coronary occlusion in acute myocardial infarction — Value of combined thrombolytic and vasodilator therapy. *N. Engl. J. Med.*, **317**, 1055–1059, 1987

20. Isner, J.M., Konstam, M.A., Fortin, R.V., *et al.* Delayed thrombolysis of streptokinase-resistant occlusive thrombus: documentation by pre- and post-mortem coronary angiography. *Am. J. Cardiol.*, **52**, 210–211, 1983

21. Waller. B.F., Rothbaum, D.A., Pinkerton, C.A., *et al.* Status of the myocardium and infarct-related coronary artery in 19 necropsy patients with acute recanalisation using pharmacologic (streptokinase, r-tissue plasminogen activator), mechanical (percutaneous transluminal coronary angioplasty) or combined types of reperfusion therapy. *J. Am. Coll. Cardiol.*, 785–801, 1987

22. Davies, M.J. Successful and unsuccessful coronary thrombolysis. *Br. Heart J.*, **61**, 381–384, 1989

23. Davies, M.J., Bland, J.M., Hangartner, J.R.W., *et al.* Factors influencing the presence or absence of acute coronary artery thrombi in sudden ischaemic death. *Eur. Heart J.*, **10**, 203–208, 1989

24. van Dantzig, J.M. and Becker, A.E. Sudden cardiac death and acute pathology of coronary arteries. *Eur. Heart J.*, **7**, 987–991, 1986

25. Davies, M.J. and Thomas, A. Thrombosis and acute coronary artery lesions in sudden cardiac ischaemic death. *N. Engl. J. Med.*, **310**, 1137–1140, 1984

26. Bruschke, A.V.G., Kramer, J.R., Bal, E.T., *et al.* The dynamics of progression of coronary atherosclerosis studied in 168 medically treated patients who underwent coronary arteriography three times. *Am. Heart J.*, **117**, 296–305, 1989

27. Richardson, P.D., Davies, M.J. and Born, G.V.R. Influence of plaque configuration and stress distribution on fissuring of coronary atherosclerotic plaques. *Lancet*, **ii**, 941–944, 1989

7

Acute myocardial infarction: a clinical view of the pathology

David Hackett

Introduction

There is now no doubt that luminal thrombosis is the fundamental process leading to and maintaining coronary occlusion in patients with acute myocardial infarction. It now seems extraordinary that there was such a doubt about the role of thrombosis over a period of 70 years, from the time of Herrick's original description in 1912 of the 'Clinical features of sudden obstruction of the coronary arteries', until the widespread application of thrombolytic therapy proved the case[1,2]. There are now substantial pathological, angiographic and angioscopic studies which demonstrate the central role of coronary arterial thrombosis in the syndrome of acute myocardial infarction[3–6]. Such thrombosis has been shown consistently to be related to plaque fissure or rupture, or with superficial endothelial damage[7,8]. What can the clinical information tell us about the underlying pathology of the coronary arteries in acute myocardial infarction?

Infarct-related coronary stenoses

In angiographic or post-mortem studies performed after myocardial infarction, but without administration of thrombolytic therapy, severely stenotic or persistently occluded coronary arteries were consistently observed[9]. These findings could not be related to the sudden onset of the syndrome in the majority of cases. When the coronary arteries are clinically examined before myocardial infarction, however, there is usually a non-obstructive stenosis present in the coronary artery supplying the infarcted area. In a study of 10 patients, who happened to have had coronary arteriography performed during a clinically stable phase of their disease before a documented myocardial infarction, we found the mean severity of obstruction of the stenosis to be 30% of diameter in the artery involved[10]. There was, however, a substantial range in severity, from 9% to 60%. And, in all but one case, these stenoses had considerably increased in severity when examined after the myocardial infarction. Two other similar studies have reported consistent findings[11,12]. These observations are compatible with the sudden, often unheralded, onset of symptoms in many cases of acute myocardial infarction. Furthermore, they also suggest that the rapid progression of coronary stenoses to become obstructive or completely occlusive is not necessarily caused by the relentless course of atherosclerotic disease, but is likely to be more consistent with the acute development of luminal thrombosis.

When thrombolytic therapy is administered to patients with acute myocardial infarction, prompt recanalization of the afflicted artery is consistently established in 50–80% of cases. The resolution of luminal thrombosis induced by thrombolytic therapy also allows us to assess the obstructive severity of pre-existing stenoses in less selected cases of acute myocardial infarction. We have examined the severity of such stenoses in a series of 60 consecutive patients presenting with their first acute myocardial infarction[13]. Using an automated, edge-detection computerized cardio-vascular angiography analysis system, the mean severity of obstruction of the residual stenoses in arteries which had become recanalized was 58%, with a range of 33–82%. A residual stenosis of less than 60% diametric obstruction was present in 47% of the patients, and one less than 50% occurred in 20% of the cases. These stenoses were even less severely obstructive after a period of 24 hours[13]. We have obtained very similar results after administration of intravenous tissue-type plasmi-nogen activator to a series of patients, and the findings are very consistent with those of Serruys *et al.*, who used similar quantitative coronary arteriographic tech-niques[14–16].

These measurements are likely to represent an overestimate of the severity of the stenoses prior to acute myocardial infarction. There may have been a variable degree of disruption by thrombosis within the plaque resulting in increased dimensions of the plaque and which was not lysed by thrombolytic agents. Not all of the luminal thrombus may have resolved early, or even late, after thrombolysis. Local and enhanced vasoconstriction may have persisted at the site of coronary arterial thrombosis (see below)[17]. These factors would all bias such assessments towards an overestimation of the severity of pre-existing stenoses in arteries supplying the zone of infarction. Nevertheless, the findings confirm that residual stenoses found after successful thrombolytic recanalization, and, therefore, also before myocardial infarction, are not necessarily severely obstructive. The findings are also consistent with the sudden onset of symptoms in most patients. Two-thirds of our cases had chest pain of sudden onset, of which one-half were completely unheralded, suggesting that most patients rapidly develop severe coronary obstruction or occlusion from mildly obstructive pre-existing stenoses[13]. This further suggests that the risk of developing arterial thrombosis and myocardial infarction is not necessarily related to the obstructive severity of pre-existing stenoses. Thus, the obstructive nature of coronary plaques in itself is not an adequate explanation for their tendency to fissure or rupture and develop luminal thrombosis. This raises the clinical problem of how to identify and manage those non-obstructive stenoses that are at risk of leading to sudden thrombotic arterial occlusion.

Coronary arterial occlusion in acute myocardial infarction

The onset of continuous chest pain is the usual clinical marker of coronary arterial occlusion in patients with acute myocardial infarction. In animal models, the rate of development of myocardial necrosis is relatively fast, and can be predicted after ligation of an artery, but, in humans, it would seem to be only poorly correlated with the duration of symptoms[18]. It is known from angiographic studies that total coronary arterial occlusion is present in 87% of patients within 4 h of the onset of symptoms, but in only 65% at 12–24 h[19]. It has previously been shown that, at 2–4 weeks after myocardial infarction, total occlusion is present in 53% of patients, and severe narrowing of the coronary artery in the remaining 47%[9]. This decline in incidence of total coronary arterial occlusion with time after the onset of symptoms in acute myocardial infarction suggests that intermittent occlusion, with transient coronary thrombosis and subsequent thrombolysis, coronary spasm, or both, may be important in the development of myocardial infarction.

We have studied the natural history of arterial occlusion in consecutive patients presenting in the early stages of acute myocardial infarction, both before and during administration of thrombolytic therapy[17]. In 36% (16 out of 45) of the patients, arteriography demonstrated recanalization and reocclusion both before and during a continuous intracoronary infusion of streptokinase. Continuous electrocardiographic monitoring demonstrated episodes of abrupt but transient and complete resolution of the ST-segment elevation to the isoelectric line in 33% (15 out of 45) of the patients, again both before and during a continuous intracoronary infusion of streptokinase. When coronary arteriography was performed during these episodes, occlusion was consistently observed during ST-segment elevation and patency during complete resolution of the ST-segment elevation.

Thus, evidence of intermittent coronary arterial occlusion was obtained by arteriography in 36% of the patients, by ST-segment monitoring before arteriography in a further 9%, and by ST-segment monitoring before the onset of chest pain in 4%. In addition, a further 20% of the patients gave a history of prolonged, discrete episodes of chest pain in the 24 hours before admission. Intermittent coronary arterial occlusion, therefore, was observed in the early stages of acute and evolving myocardial infarction in 49% of our patients, and could have been present in a total of 69% of our cases[17].

These findings have several important conclusions and implications. Dynamic occlusion of the coronary arteries might explain the intermittent nature of chest pain observed in many patients at the onset, and early in the course of, the syndrome of acute myocardial infarction. Intermittent occlusion might also explain the finding of apparently normal electrocardiograms very early in the course of acute myocardial infarction. It would also explain the poor correlation of single electrocardiographic recordings with 'spot' arteriographic findings[20]. Intermittent occlusion might explain the variations observed in ST-segment elevation detected by hourly electrocardiographic recordings in patients with acute and evolving myocardial infarction[21]. The effect of intermittent coronary arterial occlusion could have an important role in the individual variation in the rate of evolution and final extent of myocardial infarction in humans. If coronary recanalization occurs early, frequently, and is long lasting, the extent of myocardial necrosis is likely to be less than if it occurs late, rarely, and is of short duration, or else does not occur at all. The dynamic nature of coronary arterial occlusion suggests, therefore, that strategies for interventions in acute myocardial infarction should not necessarily be based only on the duration of symptoms but, perhaps, also on other indicators of the extent of myocardial necrosis such as the electrocardiographic stage of evolution of the infarction[17].

Coronary vasoconstriction

The dynamic nature of coronary arterial occlusion, both before and during continuous administration of thrombolytic therapy, suggests that pathophysiological processes other than thrombosis may be present in patients with acute myocardial infarction. We have systematically examined the responses of coronary arteries to administration of large local doses of nitrates before, during and after thrombolytic therapy in acute and evolving myocardial infarction[17,22]. An initial intracoronary dose of nitrates failed to induce patency in any case demonstrating total occlusion when arteriography was first performed. In those with initial subtotal occlusion, however, intracoronary nitrates induced prompt recanalization in 50% (three of six) of the patients. When totally occluded vessels became subtotally occluded subsequent to an infusion of streptokinase, a further intracoronary dose of nitrates promptly induced full patency in 80% (eight of ten) of the patients. When acute reocclusion was demonstrated, an intracoronary dose of nitrates induced prompt recanalization in 69% (11 of 16) of the patients. When full patency was achieved at the end of the thrombolytic procedure, a further intracoronary dose of nitrates was administered. The stenosis in the coronary artery supplying the infarcted area showed significant dilation, from 58% to 52% in obstruction diameter, whereas there was no accompanying dilatation of other adjacent, but uninvolved, normal coronary arteries.

Thus, large local doses of powerful vasodilator agents frequently relieve acute reocclusion, improve incomplete occlusion, and dilate the residual coronary arterial stenosis. These observations suggest the presence of enhanced, localized coronary vasoconstriction, possibly interacting with local thrombosis and thrombolysis, which contributes to the arterial occlusion. The failure of intracoronary nitrates to induce coronary patency before thrombolysis does not necessarily imply that coronary vasoconstriction may not be present at that stage. Nitrates may be ineffective because of inadequate concentration at the site of occlusion due to stagnation of blood flow, the presence of a large thrombotic plug, or due to the presence of powerful local constrictor stimuli at the site of an intimal lesion in close proximity to thrombus as has been demonstrated in an experimental model in laboratory animals[23,24]. At a later stage, when initial recanalization has been achieved by thrombolysis, nitrates may become effective in relieving vasoconstriction because of their delivery in adequate concentrations to the relevant segment of the coronary artery.

The extent of the dilatation achieved with nitrates is probably within the physiological range of coronary arterial tone, although the vasoconstriction has been induced by local pathological processes[25]. In patients with atypical chest pain and no atherosclerotic disease, the calibre of coronary arteries can be reduced by a mean of 16% in response to powerful constricting stimuli[26]. This is in contrast to the extreme degree of vasoconstriction observed in patients with Prinzmetal's variant angina: In such patients, with coronary spasm, the calibre of the spastic coronary artery is reduced by an average of 88% in response to constricting stimuli[26]. In patients with acute myocardial infarction, therefore, the extent of the arterial constriction and dilatation indicates that there is no evidence for the presence of that type of coronary spasm which is usually observed in cases of Prinzmetal's variant angina.

If enhanced localized vasoconstriction is present in the coronary artery supplying the infarcted zone, are vasodilator drugs useful as adjunctive therapy to thrombolytic agents in patients with acute myocardial infarction? Rentrop et al.[27] have demonstrated in a randomized controlled study that the intracoronary administration of combined streptokinase and nitroglycerin infusions to patients with early evolving myocardial infarction and total arterial occlusion resulted in a higher frequency of recanalization (19 out of 23, 83%) compared with an intracoronary infusion of streptokinase alone (13 out of 20, 65%), but these differences were not statistically significant[27]. In a second, similar, study they observed acute recanalization in 63% (39 out of 62) of the patients who received combined intracoronary infusions of streptokinase and nitroglycerin and in 60% (40 out of 67) of the cases who received streptokinase alone[28]. Again, these differences were not significantly different. If the data are pooled, they show a 7% difference (68% compared with 61%) in acute patency in favour of the adjunctive use of nitrates. In another study by Brower *et al.*[29], independent predictors of arterial patency in patients with acute myocardial infarction who received an intravenous infusion of tissue-type plasminogen activator were examined by using multivariate logistic regression analysis[29]. Patency of the coronary artery supplying the infarcted area at 90 minutes after the start of treatment was present in 72% (52 out of 72) of those cases who received combined intravenous infusions of tissue-type plasminogen activator and nitrate drugs, but in only 63% (108 out of 171) of those who received the thrombolytic agent alone. These differences were not statistically significant.

Although these studies do not demonstrate individual statistical significance, the observations do show a consistent trend towards a greater frequency of acute coronary arterial patency when a combination of systemic nitrates and thrombolytic agents are administered to patients with acute myocardial infarction. The magnitude of the differences are small, however, ranging from 7% in the pooled data of Rentrop *et al.*[27] to 9% in the larger, but non-randomized, study of Brower *et al.*[29]. Such a gain might be worthwhile in practice for a relatively simple, safe and inexpensive treatment.

Role of platelet activation and aggregation

Platelet activation is an important pathophysiological component of the syndrome of unstable angina[30,31]. Activation of platelets is also thought to be an important part of the early thrombotic response to acute plaque fissuring, particularly when considerable plaque disruption has occurred before and during the early stages of the evolving acute myocardial infarction. The administration of aspirin to patients with acute myocardial infarction has been shown to result in a reduction in mortality. This effect probably results, at least in part, from the prevention of coronary reocclusion[32]. The effect of anti-platelet agents on the specific inhibition or acute resolution of thrombosis has not, however, been systematically studied.

Prostacyclin is a powerful inhibitor of platelet aggregation and induces relaxation of vascular smooth muscle[33,34]. These actions counteract those of thromboxane A_2 released by aggregating platelets, and the net effects of prostacyclin and thromboxane A_2 may be important mechanisms in regulation of both vascular tone and the aggregation of platelets[35]. They could also be important factors in the development and maintenance of arterial occlusion in acute myocardial infarction. We, and others, have recently examined the effect of administration of prostacyclin before, during or after thrombolytic therapy in patients with acute myocardial infarction[36,37]. There was no increase in the rate of acute recanalization, or improvement in the subsequent maintenance of arterial patency, associated with the administration of prostacyclin. Furthermore, large local doses of prostacyclin did not result in consistent or significant dilatation of the acutely recanalized stenosis in the artery supplying the infarcted myocardium[37]. Thus, the use of a specific platelet anti-aggregatory agent does not seem to result in useful effects in acute myocardial infarction. This lack of consistent effect could be due to the relative inaccessibility of the intimal thrombus rich in platelets, which cannot easily be reached by such drugs in many patients. In contrast, the luminal thrombus rich in fibrin is more easily accessible but probably less responsive to intravenous, or even direct, intra-arterial administration of anti-platelet agents.

Diurnal onset of acute myocardial infarction

A diurnal pattern in the onset of acute myocardial infarction has been known for some time[38,39]. There are many biological factors that behave physiologically with circadian rhythms or diurnal variations, and which may be of possible importance in the pathogenesis of acute coronary arterial occlusion. Such factors with known diurnal variations include systemic blood pressure, heart rate, coronary blood flow, episodes of transient myocardial ischamia, platelet aggregability, levels of cortisol and adrenaline in the plasma, and tissue-type plasminogen activator[40]. We have examined the circadian patterns of the specific activities of endogenous tissue-type plasminogen activator within the plasma and its main inhibitor, the fast-acting plasminogen activator inhibitor[41].

In normal subjects, there is a considerable variation in the activity of tissue-type plasminogen activator within the plasma and its main inhibitor over a 24 hour period. The peak in activity of the activator, accompanied by the nadir in activity of the inhibitor, occurs at 15.00; while the converse nadir and peak are observed at 03.00, respectively. At 03.00, in fact, there is little endogenous fibrinolytic activity observed in most subjects. We have also observed this diurnal pattern in patients with diffuse atherosclerotic disease, and have shown that it is preserved in patients at the time of onset of acute myocardial infarction[42, 43]. It would seem reasonable to postulate that these observations have important implications regarding the pathogenesis of the thrombotic onset of acute myocardial infarction. Furthermore, the amount of free tissue-type plasminogen activator taken up by a developing thrombus is a very important determinant of the rate of fibrinolysis of that clot[44]. This diurnal variation in fibrinolytic activity, therefore, also implies that the time of day might affect the ease or difficulty with which a thrombus within a coronary artery may spontaneously lyse or resolve with administration of thrombolytic therapy.

Conclusions

Examination of the clinical information available in patients with acute myocardial infarction can provide extensive clues and implications concerning the underlying pathology, and especially the dynamic nature of many pathophysiological processes[45]. A better understanding of some of these pathophysiological processes associated with acute coronary arterial occlusion in patients with acute myocardial infarction has resulted in more specific and, therefore, probably more effective treatments. The real challenges, however, will be to identify, on a clinical rather than epidemiological basis, those patients with the greatest risk of developing acute coronary arterial thrombosis and myocardial infarction. This raises the question of how to develop clinical methods that will be able to identify and manage those patients, and the non-obstructive stenoses of their coronary arteries, which are at risk of leading to sudden thrombotic occlusion.

References

1. Herrick, J.B. Clinical features of sudden obstruction of the coronary arteries. *J. Am. Med. Assoc.*, **59**, 2015–2020, 1912
2. Laffel, G.L. and Braunwald, E. Thrombolytic therapy. A new strategy for the treatment of acute myocardial infarction. *N. Engl. J. Med.*, **311**, 710–717, 770–776, 1984
3. Davies, M.J., Woolf, N. and Robertson, W.B. Pathology of acute myocardial infarction with particular reference to occlusive coronary thrombi. *Br. Heart J.*, **38**, 659–664, 1976
4. Davies, M.J. and Thomas, A. Thrombosis and acute coronary artery lesions in sudden cardiac ischemic death. *N. Engl. J. Med.*, **310**, 1137–1140, 1984
5. DeWood, M.A., Spores, J., Notske, R., *et al.* Prevalence of total coronary occlusion during the early hours of transmural myocardial infarction. *N. Engl. J. Med.*, **303**, 897–902, 1980
6. Sherman, C.T., Litvack, F., Grundfest, W., *et al.* Coronary angioscopy in patients with unstable angina pectoris. *N. Engl. J. Med.*, **315**, 913–919, 1986
7. Falk, E. Plaque rupture with severe pre-existing stenosis precipitating coronary thrombosis. Characteristics of coronary atherosclerotic plaques underlying fatal occlusive thrombi. *Br. Heart J.*, **50**, 127–134, 1983
8. Davies, M.J. and Thomas, A.C. Plaque fissuring – the cause of acute myocardial infarction, sudden ischaemic death, and crescendo angina. *Br. Heart J.*, **53**, 363–373, 1985
9. Bertrand, M.E., Lefebvre, J.M., Laisne, C.L., *et al.* Coronary arteriography in acute transmural myocardial infarction. *Am. Heart J.*, **97**, 61–69, 1979
10. Hackett, D., Verwilghen, J., Davies, G. and Maseri, A. Coronary stenoses before and after acute myocardial infarction. *Am. J. Cardiol.*, **63**, 1517–1518, 1989
11. Ambrose, J.A., Tannenbaum, M.A., Alexopoulos, D., *et al.* Angiographic progression of coronary artery disease and the development of myocardial infarction. *J. Am. Coll. Cardiol.*, **12**, 56–62, 1988
12. Little, W.C., Constantinuescu, M., Applegate, J., *et al.* Can coronary arteriography predict the site of a subsequent myocardial infarction in patients with mild-to-moderate coronary artery disease? *Circulation*, **78**, 1157–1166, 1988
13. Hackett, D., Davies, G. and Maseri, A. Pre-existing coronary stenoses in patients with first myocardial infarction are not necessarily severe. *Eur. Heart J.*, **9**, 1317–1323, 1988
14. Khan, M., Hackett, D., McFadden, E., *et al.* Effectiveness of bolus administration of tissue-type plasminogen activator in acute myocardial infarction. *Am. J. Cardiol.*, **65**, 1051–1056, 1990
15. Serruys, P.W., Wijns, W., Van den Brand, M., *et al.* Is transluminal coronary angioplasty mandatory after successful thrombolysis? A quantitative coronary angiographic study. *Br. Heart J.*, **50**, 257–265, 1983
16. Serruys, P.W., Arnold, A.E.R., Brower, R.W., *et al.* Effect of continued rt-PA administration on the residual stenosis after initially successful recanalization in acute myocardial infarction – a quantitative coronary angiography study of a randomised trial. *Eur. Heart J.*, **8**, 1172–1181, 1987
17. Hackett, D., Davies, G., Chierchia, S. and Maseri, A. Intermittent coronary occlusion in acute myocardial infarction. Value of combined thrombolytic and vasodilator therapy. *N. Engl. J. Med.*, **317**, 1055–1059, 1987
18. Reimer, K.A., Lowe, J.E., Rasmussen, M.M. and Jennings, R.B. The wavefront phenomenon of ischemic cell death. 1. Myocardial infarct size vs duration of coronary occlusion in dogs. *Circulation*, **56**, 786–794, 1977
19. DeWood, M.A., Spores, J., Notske, R., *et al.* Prevalence of total coronary occlusion during the early hours of transmural myocardial infarction. *N. Engl. J. Med.*, **303**, 897–902, 1980
20. Bren, G.B., Wasserman, A.G. and Ross, A.M. Hazards of using post thrombolytic ST segment evolution as a reperfusion marker. Observations from the TIMI trial (abstract). *J. Am. Coll. Cardiol.*, **7**, 17A, 1986
21. Thygesen, K., Hørder, M., Nielsen, B.L. and Peterson, P.H. The variability of ST segment in the early phase of acute myocardial infarction. *Acta Med. Scand. (Suppl.)*, **623**, 61–70, 1979
22. Hackett, D., Davies, G. and Maseri, A. Coronary constriction in acute myocardial infarction – role of nitrates. *Eur. Heart J.*, **9 (Suppl. A)**, 151–153, 1988
23. Schmitz, J.M., Apprill, P.G., Buja, L.M., *et al.* Vascular prostaglandin and thromboxane production in a canine model of myocardial ischemia. *Cir. Res.*, **57**, 223–231, 1985
24. Ashton, J.H., Ogletree, M.L., Michel, I.M., *et al.* Cooperative mediation by serotonin S_2 and thromboxane A_2/prostaglandin H_2 receptor activation of cyclic flow variations in dogs with severe coronary artery stenoses. *Circulation*, **76**, 952–959, 1987
25. Maseri, A., Davies, G., Hackett, D. and Kaski, J.C. Coronary artery spasm and coronary vasoconstriction – the case for a distinction. *Circulation*, **81**, 1983–1991, 1990.

26. Hackett, D., Larkin, S., Chierchia, S., *et al.* Induction of coronary artery spasm by a direct local action of ergonovine. *Circulation,* **75,** 577–582, 1987

27. Rentrop, K.P., Feit, F., Blanke, H., *et al.* Effects of intracoronary streptokinase and intracoronary nitroglycerin infusion on coronary angiographic patterns and mortality in patients with acute myocardial infarction. *N. Engl. J. Med.,* **311,** 1457–1463, 1984

28. Rentrop, K.P., Feit, F., Sherman, W., *et al.* Late thrombolytic therapy preserves left ventricular function in patients with collateralized total coronary occlusion: primary end-point findings of the second Mount Sinai New York University Reperfusion Trial. *J. Am. Coll. Cardiol.,* **14,** 58–64, 1989

29. Brower, R.W., Arnold, A.E.R., Lubsen, J. and Verstraete, M. Coronary patency after intravenous infusion of recombinant tissue-type plasminogen activator in acute myocardial infarction. *J. Am. Coll. Cardiol.,* **11,** 681–688, 1988

30. Fitzgerald, D.J., Roy, L., Catella, R.L. and Fitzgerald, G.A. Platelet activation in unstable coronary artery disease. *N. Engl. J. Med.,* **315,** 983–989, 1986

31. Hamm, C.W., Lorenz, R.L., Bleifeld, W., *et al.* Biochemical evidence of platelet activation in patients with persistent unstable angina. *J. Am. Coll. Cardiol.,* **10,** 998–1004, 1987

32. ISIS-2 (Second International Study of Infarct Survival) Collaborative Group. Randomised trial of intravenous streptokinase, oral aspirin, both or neither among 17,187 cases of suspected acute myocardial infarction: ISIS-2. *Lancet,* **ii,** 349–360, 1988

33. Moncada, S., Gryglewski, R., Bunting, S. and Vane, J.R. An enzyme isolated from arteries transforms prostaglandin endoperoxides to an unstable substance that inhibits platelet aggregation. *Nature (Lond.),* **263,** 663–665, 1976

34. Vane, J.R. Prostaglandins and the cardiovascular system (Editorial). *Br. Heart J.,* **49,** 405–409, 1983

35. Moncada, S. and Vane, J.R. Pharmacology and endogenous roles of prostacyclin endoperoxides. thromboxane A_2, and prostacyclin. *Pharmacol. Rev.,* **30,** 293–331, 1978

36. Topol, E.J., Ellis, S.G., Califf, R.C., *et al.* and the Thrombolysis and Angioplasty in Myocardial Infarction (TAMI) 4 Study Group. Combined tissue-type plasminogen activator and prostacyclin therapy for acute myocardial infarction. *J. Am. Coll. Cardiol.,* **14,** 877–884, 1989

37. Hackett, D., Davies, G. and Maseri, A. Effect of prostacycling on coronary occlusion in acute myocardial infarction. *Int. J. Cardiol.,* **26,** 53–58, 1990

38. World Health Organization. *Myocardial Infarction Community Registers. Public Health in Europe,* vol 5, annex II, WHO, Copenhagen, pp. 188–191, 1979

39. Muller, J.E., Stone, P.H., Turi, Z.G., *et al.* and the MILIS Study Group. Circadian variation in the frequency of onset of acute myocardial infarction. *N. Engl. J. Med.,* **313,** 1315–1322, 1985

40. Muller, J.E., Tofler, G.H. and Stone, P.H. Circadian variation and triggers of onset of acute cardiovascular disease. *Circulation,* **79,** 733–743, 1989

41. Andreotti, F., Davies, G., Hackett, D., *et al.* Major circadian fluctuations in fibrinolytic factors and possible relevance to the time of onset of myocardial infarction, sudden cardiac death and stroke. *Am. J. Cardiol.,* **62,** 635–637, 1988

42. Andreotti, F., Davies, G., Hackett, D., *et al.* Circadian variation of fibrinolytic factors in normal human plasma. *Fibrinolysis,* **2 (Suppl. 2),** 90–92, 1988

43. Andreotti, F., Roncaglioni, C., Hackett, D., *et al.* Early coronary reperfusion blunts the procoagulant response of plasminogen activator inhibitor-1 and von Willibrand factor in acute myocardial infarction. *J. Am. Coll. Cardiol.,* **16,** 1553–1560, 1990

44. Brommer, E.J.P. The level of extrinsic plasminogen activator (tPA) during clotting as a determinant of the rate of fibrinolysis; inefficiency of activators added afterwards. *Thromb. Res.,* **34,** 109–115, 1984

45. Maseri, A., Chierchia, S. and Davies, G. Pathophysiology of coronary occlusion in acute infarction. *Circulation,* **73,** 233–239, 1986

8

Stratification of risk after myocardial infarction

Mark A. de Belder

Mortality rates after myocardial infarction

Of those patients admitted to hospital following a myocardial infarction, approximately 10–15% will die before the end of 2 weeks. Of the group that are discharged from hospital, the mortality rate in the first year has, until recently, been 10–20%. Thereafter, the annual mortality rate is about 5% (Figure 8.1)[1–3]. With the widespread use of thrombolytic agents, the mortality for hospital survivors within the first year should now be about 10%. Most patients who die in the first year after discharge do so in the first 6 months. Many of these patients die suddenly[4,5].

'Sudden death' is difficult to define. In many studies, all deaths within an hour of cardiac symptoms are included in the definition. A proportion of patients may die in severe cardiac failure (the terminal event in such cases may be asystole rather than a tachyarrhythmia), and a proportion may die after a fresh ischaemic insult. The terminal event in many patients, however, is sustained monomorphic ventricular

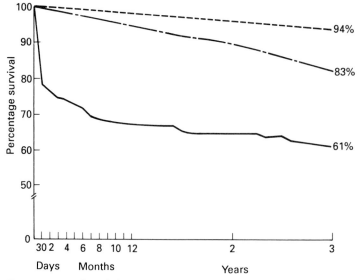

Figure 8.1 Pre-thrombolytic mortality curves following myocardial infraction. $---$ = Normal population; $-\cdot-$ = angina; $\underline{\quad\quad}$ = myocardial infarction (patients admitted to hospital). (Modified from Reference [1]).

tachycardia degenerating rapidly into ventricular fibrillation[6]. In these cases, the infarct has produced the anatomic substrate which supports a re-entry tachycardia. The tachycardia may be initiated by a number of triggers, including an appropriately timed premature ventricular contraction, increased sympathetic drive, or withdrawal of vagal tone.

Mortality thus appears to be related to three features:

1. The extent of ventricular dysfunction.
2. The presence of residual ischaemia or the possibility of a new ischaemic event.
3. The underlying tendency to arrhythmias.

The interrelations of these features are complex and will vary from patient to patient (Figure 8.2).

Need for stratification of risk

Patients can be easily stratified in terms of risk following myocardial infarction on the basis of a single investigation, such as radioisotope ventriculography. Applying this technique to all patients who are discharged from hospital (a group with a mortality over the first year of 10–20%), it is possible to identify a subgroup with an ejection fraction of 20% or less (the comparable mortality in this group is about 30%). Even though this is a group at higher risk, none the less, 70% will survive the first year. There must be factors other than the extent of ventricular damage, therefore, which distinguish those who die from those who survive. These may relate to differences in the pattern of ischaemia or the risk of arrhythmias which are independent of ventricular dysfuntion. Ideally, each of the three features described above should be evaluated in each patient.

Identification of those groups at high risk carries with it the responsibility of finding a therapeutic regimen for the individual patient which will reduce the risk of dying. Beta blackade reduces the mortality within the first year by about 20%[7]. Although these figures are favourable, further analysis demonstrates that it is somewhat optimistic to present the data in this way. If the mortality of the control group in a study is 15% within the first year, and treatment reduces the rate of mortality by 20%, then the rate of death over the first year in the group undergoing treatment would be 12%. This analysis demonstrates that, for every 100 patients treated, only three lives will be saved. The prescription of beta blockers is accepted because, although only a few patients benefit, the treatment is inexpensive and appears to do little harm to those who do not. The results of the Cardiac Arrhythmia Suppression Trial remind us that other therapies may be harmful to post-infarction patients[8]. The arguments that applied to beta blockade cannot be extrapolated to

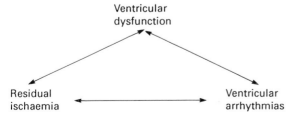

Figure 8.2 Major determinants of prognosis following myocardial infarction

other therapies which, although of major benefit to some patients, would be hazardous to others. Such therapeutic options include use of antiarrhythmic drugs, coronary arterial or ablative surgery, and implantation of cardioverter-defibrillators.

To increase the benefit-to-risk ratio for such treatments, it is essential that stratification of risk for individual end-points is as accurate as possible. A patient with poor ventricular function with no evidence of ischaemia, but who demonstrates a tendency to ventricular tachyarrhythmias, might best be treated with an implantable defibrillator. A patient with good left ventricular function and disease of all three coronary arteries might, on the other hand, be most appropriately treated with coronary arterial bypass grafting. And so on.

Predictive value of investigations and their application to large populations of patients

If a process to stratify risk is to be recommended for general use, three features must be established:

1. That the investigations involved provide additional prognostic data to that which is already available from the clinical status of the patients and from routine and simple investigations such as the 12-lead electrocardiogram and the chest X-ray. Alternatively, they must provide further insight into the pathogenic mechanisms of the end-points being investigated.
2. That the population to whom the process of stratification of risk applies is clearly defined.
3. That the process is affordable, taking into account the facilities that are available to most of the population. It should not depend on very expensive facilities available to only a minority.

The second of these features is particularly important and must be considered in relation to the third. Bayes' theorem reminds us that the predictive value of a test will depend on the prior probability of the disease (or end-point) undergoing study in the population being investigated. The prior probability of death in the first year for all survivors of myocardial infarction who leave hospital is 10–20%. That for the subgroup with an ejection fraction of 20% or less is about 30%. The predictive value of a single investigation might, thus, be expected to differ when applied to these different groups of patients. A practical application of this theorem to survivors of infarction is to use a preliminary screening test which is sensitive, but not necessarily specific, for mortality. This preliminary investigation, which should be widely available, cheap, and easy to apply, is then used as a screening test to select out a group at higher risk. The smaller group at higher risk can then be referred to centres with more expensive but more specific investigations. By applying a series of tests, it may be possible to identify a group with a very high mortality during the first year. Such a group would be the most appropriate to study so as to evaluate the benefits of certain therapies.

Methods of investigating patients

The traditional and more novel methods of quantifying the three features described above are listed in Table 8.1.

Table 8.1 Investigations for stratification of risk following myocardial infarction

	Left ventricular dysfunction	Ischaemic risk	Potential for arrhythmias
Non-invasive	Clinical features 12-lead ECG Chest X-ray Cardiac enzymes Echocardiography Exercise testing Radionuclide ventriculography MR imaging	Clinical features 12-lead ECG Ambulatory ECG (ST analysis) Exercise testing Radionuclide perfusion studies Stress echocardiography MR imaging Positron emission scintigraphy	Clinical features 12-lead ECG Telemetry Ambulatory ECG (arrhythmia analysis) Exercise testing Signal-averaged ECG Autonomic function tests – 1 – heart rate variability
Invasive	Angiography	Arteriography	Autonomic function tests – 2 – baroreceptor sensitivity test Programmed electrical stimulation

ECG = electrocardiogram; MR = magnetic resonance.

Extent of left ventricular dysfunction

The extent of left ventricular dysfunction can be assessed clinically, aided by features of the 12-lead electrocardiogram and the chest X-ray. These are fairly crude methods, enabling only the broadest stratification of patients (for example, anterior as opposed to inferior infarction; non-Q wave versus Q wave infarction; Killip class I–IV, see Table 8.2), and so on [9]. More precise quantification can be achieved by measuring cardiac enzymes, although the timing of sampling blood from the onset of infarction (often difficult to define) is important. Other relatively simple investigations include echocardiography, exercise testing and radionuclide ventriculography. Many studies have used the results of left ventricular cine-angiography combined with coronary arteriography. Digital subtraction techniques with intravenous injection of contrast can also be used. Magnetic resonance imaging also measures the extent of ventricular dysfunction, but it is expensive and available at present in only a few centres.

Continuing ischaemic risk

Continuing ischaemic risk is sometimes obvious clinically, but, for the asymptomatic patient, features of the 12-lead electrocardiogram (e.g. non-Q wave infarction) and other electrocardiographic investigations are useful. These include exercise testing and analysis of the ST segment following ambulatory monitoring. Other methods of investigation include radionuclide perfusion scans and stress imaging, whether with echocardiography, magnetic resonance or positron emission scintigraphy. Although many non-invasive methods have replaced the need to proceed to left ventriculography in cardiac patients in general, no non-invasive investigation has replaced coronary arteriography for the assessment of coronary arterial anatomy.

Potential for arrhythmias

Non-invasive methods of assessing the potential for arrhythmias include clinical status and electrocardiography (single and 12-lead, single lead monitoring during the first 24–48 h, telemetry during the convalescent period, ambulatory recordings, exercise testing, and more recently, signal-averaged electrocardiography). Newer methods include an assessment of the variability of heart-rate and, more invasively,

Table 8.2 Stratification of risk following myocardial infarction – Killip classes

	Killip class			
	I No CHF	II CHF	III Pulmonary oedema	IV Cardiogenic shock
Distribution in patients	33%	38%	10%	19%
Proportion with life-threatening arrhythmias	36%	46%	73%	94%
Incidence of cardiac arrest	5%	15%	46%	77%
Hospital mortality	6%	17%	38%	81%

Modified from Killip and Kimball [9]
CHF = congestive heart failure.

study of the sensitivity of baroreceptor reflexes and programmed electrical stimulation of the ventricles.

Choice of investigations – traditional methods

Faced with this barrage of tests, it is not surprising that different groups have used different approaches for the stratification of risk, depending on the facilities and expertise that are available. For a protocol to be widely applied to a large population scattered across the country, the initial process of stratification should depend on a combination of clinical acumen and a few widely available and simple investigations.

Prognostic indices

It must first be established whether anything more is needed beyond the clinical evaluation of the patient, the 12-lead electrocardiogram and the chest X-ray. As demonstrated in Table 8.2, Killip and Kimball[9] were able to stratify their patients subsequent to myocardial infarction on the basis of varying degrees of heart failure. This classification is also useful for long-term stratification. Variables derived from the clinical status of the patient and the electrocardiogram formed the basis of the coronary prognostic index developed by Peel and colleagues[10]. The more widely used index developed by Norris and colleagues also used features of the chest X-ray[11–13]. Multivariable analysis was performed on a large number of variables to identify those giving the most prognostic information. Scores are given to patients on the basis of the following:

1. Their age.
2. The position and type of infarct as determined electrocardiographically.
3. The systolic blood pressure at the time of admission.
4. The size of the heart on the chest X-ray.
5. The appearances of the lung fields on the chest X-ray.
6. A previous history of angina or infarction.

The total score is used to stratify patients, as shown in Figure 8.3. These, and other prognostic indices, are, perhaps, most useful in stratifying the patients at the very highest risk, and are less powerful in stratifying the majority of patients who undergo an uncomplicated recovery. In addition, they do not provide data about the likely mode of death, and thus are not useful in determining the most appropriate therapy for the individual patient.

It is likely (although still not proven) that many patients will benefit from revascularization after a myocardial infarction. If this is so, and because there is no alternative to coronary arteriography (which is routinely performed with left ventricular cine-angiography), it could be argued that many of the other investigations become redundant in the assessment of such patients. They may help, however, in determining which patients should be investigated by angiography. Patients with severe pump failure, those with continuing ischaemic pain following infarction, and those who suffer a ventricular tachyarrhythmia in the late convalescent phase (after 2 days) are all at higher risk of dying and should be investigated with angiography. There is no need to submit all those patients who are clinically stable to angiography because many of them will have a good prognosis. The non-invasive tests can be applied to this group.

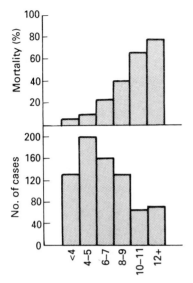

Figure 8.3 Use of the Norris Coronary Prognostic Index (CPI) in determining hospital mortality of patients following myocardial infarction. Modified from reference[10]

Although it has been suggested that radionuclide studies are more sensitive in detecting patients at high risk than are other investigations[14], they are expensive and demand expertise in interpretation. Exercise testing is available in nearly all hospitals and provides important information, not only on the likelihood of future ischaemic events, but also on the extent of ventricular dysfunction and the potential for arrhythmias. The development of any one of a number of variables should thus be used to define an abnormal test (Table 8.3).

Importance of exercise testing[15–17]

ST segment depression of at least 0.1 mV developing in any lead, measured 80 ms after the J point, indicates a continuing risk of ischaemia, whether associated with angina or not. Down-sloping ST segment depression is suggestive of triple vessel disease[18]. Elevation of the ST segment has been shown in most studies to be associated with the extent of left ventricular dysfunction, although, in certain

Table 8.3 Variables defining an abnormal exercise test following myocardial infarction

ST segment depression
Development of angina
Abnormal blood pressure responses*
Stopping at low work-load*
Development of ventricular arrhythmias*

and possibly

ST segment elevation
Development of supraventricular arrhythmias*

*Variably defined.

patients, it may indicate a continuing risk of ischaemia. Its inclusion in the list of variables defining a positive test makes the exercise test more sensitive, but less specific, for clinical end-points[17]. An abnormal response by blood pressure is a particularly useful marker of higher risk of dying in the first year. Although this is defined in many ways in the literature, a failure of the systolic blood pressure to rise by 10 mm Hg, or having risen, to fall again by 10 mm Hg or more, has been demonstrated to identify a group at high risk using a submaximal exercise protocol. Another important variable in determining the risk of dying in the first year is the development of ventricular arrhythmias. These are also defined in many ways, but in general include a count of premature ventricular contractions of between 6 and 10 per minute during or after exercise, or the development of couplets, triplets, or longer salvos.

Two questions that have not yet been fully resolved concern the most appropriate exercise protocol and its timing after infarction. Those who advocate a maximal exercise test performed later after infarction (at 4–6 weeks) suggest that this protocol is more sensitive for the detection of patients at higher risk than is an earlier (pre-discharge) submaximal test. A later test, however, will 'miss' a not insignificant minority of patients at high risk who will die within the first 4–6 weeks. In addition, a pre-discharge test is easier to organize logistically, is useful in identifying and encouraging patients at low risk, and identifies subgroups of patients at very high risk who should be further investigated sooner rather than later. Some centres are now using pre-discharge maximal (i.e. symptom-limited) protocols, while others use a submaximal protocol at 3 days for selected patients deemed to be of low risk, thus identifying a group who can be safely discharged within the first week of infarction. The exact details of such a protocol are not that important, but each centre should know the prognostic information that its selected protocol provides.

Patients with a normal ('negative') exercise test have a good prognosis, with a mortality rate of between 0.5 and 4% over the first year. It could be argued that these patients should be encouraged, do not need any further investigations, should be rapidly rehabilitated, and may not need protection with secondary preventive therapeutic agents. Patients with an abnormal ('positive') test have an overall mortality of 15–25% within the first year and should be investigated further.

It is suggested, then, that patients can be stratified initially on the basis of their clinical status and the results of an exercise test. Of those patients who are clinically stable following infarction, about half will have a positive exercise test. The vast majority of patients who will die in the first year will be identified by their early clinical features and an abnormal result from their exercise test. Although this combination is sensitive in identifying high-risk patients, however, it is not very specific.

Ambulatory Holter recordings and radionuclide ventriculography[19–21]

The detection of both supraventricular and ventricular arrhythmias in convalescent patients after myocardial infarction has been simplified by the automated analysis of ambulatory electrocardiograms. The arrhythmias detected can be classified in a number of ways. The average hourly count of premature contractions is one simple means of stratifying patients. A count of 10 or more per hour is associated with a mortality within the first year of at least 15%. This classification is very simple and does not take into account the number and frequency of other arrhythmias, such as ventricular couplets, salvos of ventricular tachycardia and so on. Lown has suggested a more complex classification of arrhythmias on these recordings which can be applied to patients suffering myocardial infarction (Table 8.4)[21].

The combination of Holter recordings and radionuclide ventriculography has been used in several large studies to identify a group of patients at relatively high risk. These studies have used the count of premature contractions together with the ejection fraction to classify patients. Mortality rates in the first year increase exponentially with falling ejection fraction (Figure 8.4). Patients with an ejection fraction of less than 30%, who also have complex ventricular arrhythmias, have a mortality of over 40% within 2 years. On the grounds that it is desirable to know the coronary arterial anatomy of high-risk patients, and that high-risk patients can be identified on clinical grounds and exercise testing, it can be argued that there is no need for radionuclide studies. These might best be reserved for patients who are unable to exercise. Those who are unable to exercise because of their cardiac status are a group at particularly high risk; mortality in the first year is 40–50%. These patients should probably proceed directly to angiography. Those who are unable to exercise because of physical disabilities (such as arthritis) can be studied with radioisotope techniques using other forms of stress (such as intravenous dipyridamole).

Table 8.4 Lown grading of ambulatory electrocardiograms[21]

Lown grade	Finding
0	Normal
1	Infrequent unifocal PVCs' (<30/h)
2	Frequent unifocal PVCs' (>30/h)
3	Multiform PVCs'
4a	Couplets present
4b	Triplets or salvos
5	Early (R-on-T) PVC's

PVC = Premature ventricular contraction.

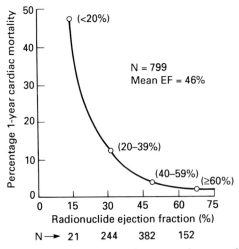

Figure 8.4 First-year mortality rate and ejection fraction. Modified from reference[19]

The identification of premature contractions on Holter recordings might be a sensitive method of identifying patients at higher risk, but this test also lacks specificity, and its positive predictive accuracy is low. These recordings might be useful, however, in selecting which patients are most appropriately investigated with other techniques (see below).

Left ventriculography and coronary arteriography[17,22,23]

An analysis of the left ventricular angiogram provides a good method of assessing the extent of left ventricular dysfunction. The procedure is used to measure the left ventricular end-diastolic pressure, to assess abnormalities of regional wall motion, and to calculate the ejection fraction. Both this, and coronary arteriography, have been shown to enhance the stratification of risk based on clinical features and exercise testing. The latter feature helps to identify those who might fare better with revascularization than with medical therapy. Patients with triple vessel disease have a worse prognosis than those with single vessel disease, although prognosis for each group is still determined primarily by the extent of ventricular dysfunction.

Newer approaches

If these investigations are limited, it is because they remain fairly non-specific in identifying those who are at risk of sudden death. More recent methods have concentrated on determining the arrhythmic potential of the patient. Holter recordings and exercise testing both have relatively low predictive accuracy, but they are also limited because they are more useful in identifying triggers of malignant ventricular arrhythmias than the substrate needed to sustain them. The newer techniques have been aimed at identifying patients with the substrate for these events. A combination of investigations that identify an underlying substrate and likely triggers of events might provide a powerful means of stratification of risk in these patients.

Signal-averaged surface electrocardiography[24–28]

The QRS complex of the surface electrocardiogram is a summation of electrical activity during ventricular depolarization. In studies using endocardial and epicardial electrodes in patients with ischaemic heart disease who were prone to sustained ventricular tachycardia, low-amplitude electrical activity was observed immediately following ventricular depolarization. This activity was observed immediately following ventricular depolarization. This activity may be a 'bystander' phenomenon, but is generally regarded as being associated with the underlying substrate for a re-entry tachycardia. The areas of delayed depolarization responsible for these arrhythmias are small in mass and produce body surface electrical potentials in the microvolt range. This activity can be detected with high-gain amplifiers, which lead inevitably to a great deal of noise. Noise reduction can be achieved by the technique of signal-averaging together with low- and high-pass filtering.

There are several different methodologies and definitions of these low-amplitude 'late potentials' which, unfortunately, do not correlate well. The most commonly used computer-assisted method is that described by Simson using the three Frank orthogonal electrode leads[24]. One or two hundred beats are acquired before the noise falls to a satisfactory level. The three orthogonal signals are averaged after amplification and filtering, and a combined vector magnitude is calculated by taking the square root of the sums of the squares of the individual vectors of the three leads (the root mean square). The noise level of the ST segment is determined and the end of the QRS is defined as the point at which the root mean square voltage is more than 2.5 times greater than the noise level. Three parameters are then measured:

1. The root mean square of the voltage over the last 40 ms of the signal-averaged complex (the RMS40).
2. The duration of high frequency potentials of less than 40 μV at the end of the QRS complex (the LPD40).
3. The total duration of the signal-averaged QRS complex.

With this method, the presence of late potentials depends on the presence of at least two of the following definitions (patients with bundle branch block excluded) (Figure 8.5):

1. A filtered QRS duration of 120 ms or more.
2. A duration of the filtered QRS after its amplitude falls below 40 μV of 40 ms or more.
3. A root mean square voltage during the last 40 ms of less than 25 μV.

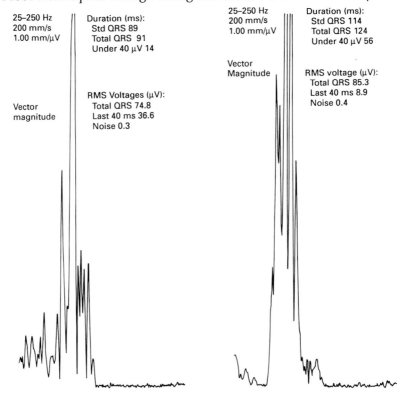

Figure 8.5. Signal-averaged electrocardiogram of (a) a survivor following myocardial infarction with no late potentials present, and (b) a patient who has been resuscitated in the late convalescent phase following infarction, demonstrating the presence of late potentials. In (b), the LPD40 (see text) is 56 ms and the root mean square (RMS) voltage during the last 40 ms is 8.9 μV.

Using such criteria, several groups have reported on the prognostic significance of late potentials in post-infarct patients. In general, they provide a relatively sensitive marker for future arrhythmic events (sustained ventricular tachycardia and sudden death) but the specificity is low as up to 40% of survivors of infarction have late potentials. The technique may be of value either in enhancing the predictive accuracy of other techniques for detection of clinical end-points (such as ejection fraction), or in determining which patients should undergo programmed electrical stimulation.

Programmed electrical stimulation of the ventricles [29–32]

Programmed electrical stimulation of the ventricle is a very useful technique for the study of patients with ventricular tachyarrhythmias. The clinical arrhythmia can be induced in nearly all patients with sustained monomorphic ventricular tachycardia. A right ventricular pacing electrode is positioned transvenously at the right ventricular apex or outflow tract and paced extrastimuli are delivered first in sinus rhythm and then at several rates during paced rhythm.

There have now been 13 major studies in which this technique has been applied to survivors of myocardial infarction. The hypothesis being tested in these studies was that the induction of a ventricular tachyarrhythmia reveals the substrate for such an arrhythmia, and points to a pathogenic mechanism of sudden death which could then be used to guide specific treatment. There has been considerable disagreement, however, about the role of this technique. The apparent discrepancy between studies is due to major differences in the stimulation protocols used and the risk status of the patients undergoing investigation. In addition, many of the studies have been too small, with an insufficient period of follow-up to demonstrate the prognostic information that can be derived. The consensus from the more recent and larger

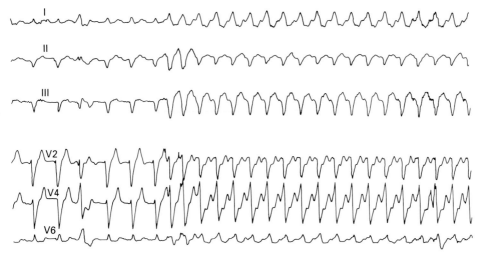

Figure 8.6. Induction of sustained monomorphic ventricular tachycardia in a survivor of myocardial infarction. The surface electrocardiographic leads shown are (from top to bottom) I, II, III, V2, V4, V6. The patient has left bundle branch block and first degree heart block during sinus rhythm. The sequence shown is as follows: two sinus beats, a ventricular extrasystole, three sinus beats, two paced premature extrastimuli followed by sustained monomorphic ventricular tachycardia (paper speed 25 mm/s).

studies is that the induction of sustained monomorphic ventricular tachycardia is one of the most accurate predictors of sudden death or the development of the same arrhythmia in the first year (Figure 8.6).

There is a need for standardization of the stimulation protocol. Some studies have used a very 'aggressive' protocol. These may be appropriate when applied to patients who have already presented with a ventricular tachyarrhythmia, but their application in a screening programme to patients who have not suffered such a clinical event needs further assessment. Stimulation at the right ventricular outflow tract, or even in the left ventricle, is not advocated for patients who have never spontaneously experienced a ventricular tachyarrhythmia. The protocol recommended is based on the protocol proposed by Wellens and his colleagues[33] (Table 8.5) with stimulation only at the right ventricular apex. The protocol should only be terminated prematurely if a sustained ventricular tachyarrhythmia is induced. Unfortunately, the more aggressive the protocol, the more likely it is that polymorphic ventricular tachycardia or fibrillation is induced. With the later stages of the protocol of Wellens et al., about 35% of all patients will develop one of these responses. Unfortunately, they do not appear to have any prognostic use. It may be that terminating the protocol with the development of non-sustained polymorphic responses in the last four stages of the protocol will reduce the incidence of these troublesome arrhythmias without reducing the sensitivity of the technique for identifying those with a substrate for sustained monomorphic ventricular tachycardia.

A further analysis of these studies reveals that the induction of sustained tachycardia is more likely in higher risk patients. Because patients with a negative exercise test have a good prognosis, I advocate that these patients do not need to undergo this investigation, which is invasive and labour intensive. All patients with a positive exercise test, and patients identified to be at high risk on clinical grounds, should be considered for this technique. This would mean recommending the technique for 50–60% of all survivors, which is probably inappropriate. Some of the other non-invasive investigations might be useful in selecting patients for programmed stimulation. There is a relatively strong correlation between those with late potentials and the inducibility of sustained monomorphic ventricular tachycardia, but if this alone was used, programmed stimulation would still be recommended for 40%

Table 8.5 Suggested stimulation protocol for survivors of myocardial infarction[33]

Stage	Basic rhythm	No. of extrastimuli
1	Sinus	1
2	Sinus	2
3	V pacing 100 bpm	1
4	V pacing 100 bpm	2
5	V pacing 120 bpm	1
6	V pacing 120 bpm	2
7	V pacing 140 bpm	1
8	V pacing 140 bpm	2
9	Sinus	3
10	V pacing 100 bpm	3
11	V pacing 120 bpm	3
12	V pacing 140 bpm	3

V = Ventricular; bpm = beats per minute.

of patients. The combination of late potentials and other factors (such as a positive exercise test, the development of non-sustained or sustained tachycardia on a Holter recording, and so on) might narrow down the selection of patients without reducing the predictive accuracy of programmed stimulation.

Autonomic function tests [34–38]

Although the mechanisms are not entirely clear, some patients demonstrate an imbalance between parasympathetic and sympathetic influences on the heart following infarction. Patients with inferior infarction, for example, are prone to pronounced vagally mediated bradycardia due to stimulation of chemoreceptors in the infero-posterior region of the left ventricle. The observation that altered autonomic activity may have prognostic implications was first made by Wolf *et al.* [34], who noted that a loss of sinus arrhythmia on admission was associated with a worse in-hospital prognosis. Since then, several groups have developed automatic techniques to measure variability in heart-rate from Holter recordings. A number of statistical indices can be used to describe the loss of such variability. These methods have been shown, in some recent studies, to be a good predictor of sudden death following myocardial infarction. The loss of variability is associated in patients at high risk with loss of vagal activity and predominant sympathetic activity. More work is needed in this area before the sensitivity and specificity of the technique is determined.

Another potentially useful investigation measures arterial baroreceptor sensitivity. The rise in arterial blood pressure secondary to intravenous phenylephrine is measured. This is normally associated with a reflex slowing of the heart rate. Baroreceptor sensitivity is expressed as the gradient of the least fit linear regression line relating the change in systolic pressure to the change in RR interval (Figure 8.7). Patients with a reduced sensitivity have been shown to be more prone to ventricular tachyarrhythmias. Recently, in a relatively small study, 90% of patients with sustained monomorphic ventricular tachycardia induced by programmed stimulation had a baroreceptor sensitivity less than 3 ms/mm Hg [38]. This suggests that this investigation may be useful in identifying patients who should undergo programmed stimulation.

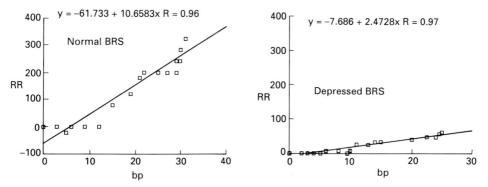

Figure 8.7. Baroreceptor sensitivity (BRS) expressed as the gradient of the least fit linear regression line derived from a plot of change in systolic pressure (in mmHg) vs change in RR interval (in ms) following an intravenous injection of phenylephrine. In plot (a), the patient is an uncomplicated survivor of infarction; in (b) a reduced BRS is found in a patient in whom sustained monomorphic ventricular tachycardia was induced with programmed electrical stimulation of the right ventricle.

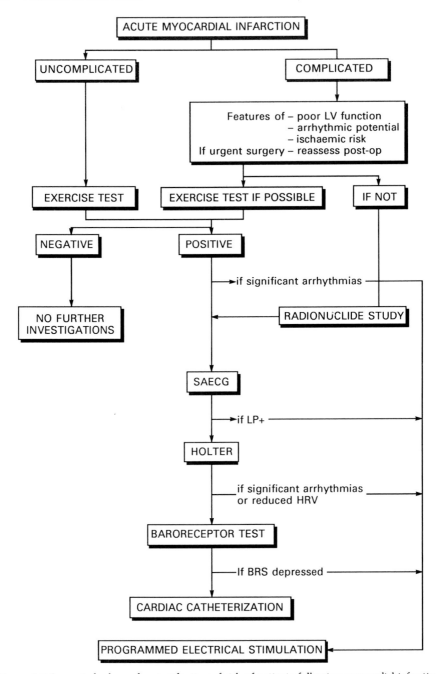

Figure 8.8 Suggested scheme for stratification of risk of patients following myocardial infarction. LV = Left ventricular; SAECG = signal averaged electrocardiogram; LP = late potential; HRV = heart rate variability; BRS = baroreceptor sensitivity

Conclusions

With our present knowledge, a suggested scheme for stratitification of risk following infarction is outlined in Figure 8.8. Such a scheme attempts to determine the extent of ventricular dysfunction, the residual ischaemic risk and the arrhythmogenic potential of each patient. It uses a simple screening test initially to identify a group at higher risk who can be studied further with more sophisticated investigations. Patients who have a complicated course following infarction, and those with a positive exercise test, should be investigated with angiography. The definition of a positive exercise test requires more than the development of ST segment shifts or angina. Development of ventricular arrhythmias, an abnormal blood pressure response, or termination of exercise at a low work-load should be included. Those who are at particular risk of future arrhythmic events, identified by a series of tests (signal-averaged and ambulatory electrocardiogram, and possibly tests of autonomic function) should be investigated by programmed electrical stimulation of the ventricle.

Patients should be stratified not only for sudden death, but also for other clinical end-points such as recurrent infarction and progressive cardiac failure. The predictive power of the investigations must be clearly understood by appropriate Bayesian analysis. With these techniques, groups at high risk with an expected first-year mortality of 40% and above can be identified. These patients are the most appropriate for studies of new secondary preventive therapies. Stratification of risk using these techniques is particularly important in the era of thrombolysis, as identifying the patients at high risk will become more of a challenge.

Acknowledgements

I am very grateful to Dr T. Farrell, St. George's Hospital Medical School, for providing Figures 8.5–8.7.

References

1. Henning, H., Gilpin, E.A., Covell, J.W., *et al.* Prognosis after myocardial infarction: a multivariate analysis of mortality and survival. *Circulation*, **59**, 1124–1136, 1979
2. Kannel, W.E., Sorlie, P. and McNamara, P.M. Prognosis after initial myocardial infarction: the Framingham Study. *Am. J. Cardiol.*, **44**, 53–59, 1979
3. Davis, H.T., DeCamilla, J., Bayer, L.W. and Moss, A.J. Survivorship patterns in the posthospital phase of myocardial infarction. *Circulation*, **60**, 1252–1258, 1979
4. Bigger, J.T., Jr., Heller, C.A., Wenger, T.L. and Weld, F.M. Risk stratification after acute myocardial infarction. *Am. J. Cardiol.*, **42**, 202–210, 1978
5. Marcus, F.I., Cobb, L.A., Edwards, J.E., *et al.*, and the Multicenter Postinfarction Research Group. Mechanisms of death and prevalence of myocardial ischemic symptoms in the terminal event after acute myocardial infarction. *Am. J. Cardiol.*, **61**, 8–15, 1988
6. Norris, R.M. and Sammel, N.L. Predictors of late hospital death in acute myocardial infarction. *Prog. Cardiovasc. Dis.*, **23**, 129–140, 1980
7. Yusuf, S., Peto, R., Lewis, J., *et al.* Beta blockade during and after myocardial infarction: an overview of the randomised trials. *Prog. Cardiovasc. Dis.*, **27**, 335–371, 1985
8. The Cardiac Arrhythmia Suppression Trial (CAST) Investigators. Preliminary report: effect of encainide and flecainide on mortality in a randomized trial of arrhythmia suppression after myocardial infarction. *N. Engl. J. Med.*, **321**, 406–412, 1989
9. Killip, T. and Kimball, J.T. Treatment of myocardial infarction in a coronary care unit. A two year experience with 250 patients. *Am. J. Cardiol.*, **20**, 457–464, 1967

10. Peel, A.A.F., Semple, T., Wang, I., et al. A coronary prognostic index for grading the severity of infarction. Br. Heart J., **25**, 745–760, 1962
11. Norris, R.M., Brandt, P.W.T., Caughey, D.E., et al. A new coronary prognostic index. Lancet, **i**, 274–278, 1969
12. Norris, R.M., Brandt, P.W.T. and Lee, A.J. Mortality in a coronary-care unit analysed by a new coronary prognostic index. Lancet, **i**, 278–281, 1969
13. Norris, R.M., Caughey, D.E., Deeming, L.W., et al. Coronary prognostic index for predicting survival after recovery from acute myocardial infarction. Lancet, **ii**, 485–487, 1970
14. Gibson, R.S., Watson, D.D., Craddock, G.B., et al. Prediction of cardiac events after uncomplicated myocardial infarction: a prospective study comparing predischarge exercise thallium-201 scintigraphy and coronary angiography. Circulation, **68**, 321–336, 1983
15. Theroux, P., Waters, D.D., Halphen, C., et al. Prognostic value of exercise testing soon after myocardial infarction. N. Engl. J. Med., **301**, 341–345, 1979
16. Weld, F.M., Chu, K-L., Bigger, J.T., Jr. and Rolnitzky, L.M. Risk stratification with low-level exercise testing 2 weeks after acute myocardial infarction. Circulation, **64**, 306–314, 1981
17. de Belder, M.A., Pumphrey, C.W., Skehan, J.D., et al. Relative power of clinical, exercise test, and angiographic variables in predicting clinical outcome after myocardial infarction: the Newham and Tower Hamlets study. Br. Heart J., **60**, 377–389, 1988
18. Mannering, D., Bennett, B.D., Ward, D.E., et al. Accurate detection of triple vessel disease in patients with exercise induced ST segment depression after infarction. Br. Heart J., **57**, 133–138, 1987
19. The Multicenter Postinfarction Research Group. Risk stratification and survival after myocardial infarction. N. Engl. J. Med., **309**, 331–336, 1983
20. Mukharji, J., Rude, R.E., Poole, K., et al. and the MILIS Study Group. Risk factors for sudden death after acute myocardial infarction: two year follow-up. Am. J. Cardiol., **54**, 31–36, 1984
21. Lown, B. and Wolf, M. Approaches to sudden death from coronary heart disease. Circulation, **44**, 130–142, 1971
22. Sanz, G., Castaner, A., Betriu, A., et al. Determinants of prognosis in survivors of myocardial infarction. A prospective clinical angiographic study. N. Engl. J. Med., **306**, 1065–1070, 1982
23. Schulman, S.P., Achuff, S.C., Griffith, L.S.C., et al. Prognostic cardiac catheterization variables in survivors of acute myocardial infarction: a five year prospective study. J. Am. Coll. Cardiol., **11**, 1164–1172, 1988
24. Simson, M.B. Use of signals in the terminal QRS complex to identify patients with ventricular tachycardia after myocardial infarction. Circulation, **64**, 235–242, 1981
25. Breithardt, G. and Borgreffe, M. Pathophysiological mechanisms and clinical significance of ventricular late potentials. Eur. Heart J., **7**, 364–385, 1986
26. Kuchar, D.L., Thorburn, C.W. and Sammel, N.L. Prediction of serious arrhythmic events after myocardial infarction: signal averaged electrocardiogram, Holter monitoring and radionuclide ventriculography. J. Am. Coll. Cardiol., **9**, 531–538, 1987
27. Cripps, T., Bennett, D., Camm, J. and Ward, D. Prospective evaluation of clinical assessment, exercise testing and signal-averaged electrocardiogram in predicting outcome after acute myocardial infarction. Am. J. Cardiol., **62**, 995–999, 1988
28. Gomes, J.A., Winters, S.L., Martinson, M., et al. The prognostic significance of quantatitive signal-averaged variables relative to clinical variables, site of myocardial infarction, ejection fraction and ventricular premature beats: a prospective study. J. Am. Coll. Cardiol., **13**, 377–384, 1989
29. Richards, D.A., Cody, D.V., Denniss, A.R., et al. Ventricular electrical instability: a predictor of death after myocardial infarction. Am. J. Cardiol., **51**, 75–80, 1983
30. Denniss, A.R., Baaijens, H., Cody, D.V., et al. Value of programmed stimulation and exercise testing in predicting one-year mortality after acute myocardial infarction. Am. J. Cardiol., **56**, 213–220, 1985
31. Waspe, L.E., Seinfield, D., Ferrick, A., et al. Prediction of sudden death and spontaneous ventricular tachycardia in survivors of complicated myocardial infarction: value of the response to programmed stimulation using a maximum of three ventricular extrastimuli. J. Am. Coll. Cardiol., **5**, 1292–1301, 1985
32. de Belder, M.A., Risk Stratification Following Myocardial Infarction: a Protocol Using Exercise Testing, Angiography and Programmed Electrical Stimulation of the Right Ventricle, MD Thesis, University of London, 1990
33. Wellens, H.J.J., Brugada, P. and Stevenson, W.G. Programmed electrical stimulation: its role in the management of ventricular arrhythmias in coronary heart disease. Prog. Cardiovasc. Dis., **29**, 165–180, 1986
34. Wolf, M.W., Varigos, G.A., Hunt, D. and Sloman, J.G. Sinus arrhythmia in acute myocardial infarction. Med. J. Austr., **2**, 52–53, 1978

35. Kleiger, R.E., Miller, J.F., Bigger, J.T., Jr., Moss, A.J., and the Multicenter Postinfarction Research Group. Decreased heart rate variability and its association with increased mortality after acute myocardial infraction. *Am. J. Cardiol.*, **59,** 256–262, 1987
36. Cripps, T.R. *A Critical Evaluation of Novel Approaches to Risk Stratification in Patients Convalescent after Acute Myocardial Infarction.* DM Thesis, University of Oxford, 1989
37. La Rovere, M.T., Specchia, G., Mortara, A. and Schwartz, P.J. Baroreflex sensitivity, clinical correlates and cardiovascular mortality among patients with a first myocardial infarction. A prospective study. *Circulation*, **78,** 816–824, 1988
38. Farrell, T.G., Cripps, T.C., Paul, V. and Camm, A.J. Baroreceptor sensitivity in patients after infarction: correlation with electrophysiological studies. *Br. Heart J.*, **61,** 472–473 (abstract), 1989

9

Invasive treatment of acute myocardial infarction

Miles Williams and Ulrich Sigwart

Introduction

The past 10 years have been witness to major changes in the treatment of both ischaemic heart disease and acute myocardial infraction. The introduction of different strategies for reperfusion finally offered a means by which the natural history of infarction could be improved, with preservation of myocardial function and reduction in mortality. Large-scale trials were implemented quickly, designed to detect differences in mortality between patients randomized to thrombolytic therapy as opposed to conventional treatment. The results were unequivocally in favour of thrombolysis[1–4]. But, questions remained regarding other parameters, such as the success rate of recanalization[5–7], the timing of reperfusion[8,9], and the preservation of left ventricular function[10–12]. It became clear that there existed a subset of patients who failed to benefit from thrombolysis, or did not derive as great a benefit as expected[7,13,14]. And there were those patients in whom thrombolysis was contraindicated[14]. Identifying such patients, and providing an alternative treatment, has become a major goal of the 'interventionists'. Researchers have focused on the role of coronary agiography and percutaneous transluminal coronary angioplasty in the context of acute myocardial infarction. When should angioplasty be used in preference to, or in association with, thrombolytic therapy, and when is it too late to attempt to achieve reperfusion? The purpose of this chapter is to review current trends in the integration of thrombolysis, coronary angiography and coronary angioplasty. The strategies of 'direct', 'immediate' and 'rescue' angioplasty will be examined.

Background

The observations of De Wood and his colleagues, published in 1980[15], were instrumental in changing the approach to myocardial infarction. Between 1971 and 1978, 322 patients were evaluated by coronary angiography and ventriculography within 24 h of onset of the symptoms of transmural infarction. The patients were separated into four discrete groups, reflecting the interval from the onset of symptoms to evaluation by arteriography. The subsets were not notably different in terms of mean age, sex, area of infarction or clinical classification on entry into the study. The paper highlighted four major points:

1. That coronary angiography could be performed safely in the setting of developing myocardial infarction (subsequently established by a large number of prospective angiographic trials).
2. That the early period (up to 4 h) of transmural infarction is characterized by total occlusion of the vessel feeding the infarcted area (in 87.3% of cases) and that the occurrence of total occlusion remains high (85.3% at 4–6 h after the onset of symptoms.
3. There is a spontaneous rate of recanalization (either due to dissolution of thrombus or to resolution of coronary arterial spasm) so that the incidence of complete occlusion falls to approximately 65% between 12 and 24 h after the onset of symptoms.
4. Patients with cardiogenic shock are more likely to have total occlusion throughout the 24 h period of study than are those who do not manifest shock.

Prior to the introduction of thrombolysis, the in-hospital prognosis for patients suffering from an acute myocardial infarction had been well defined in numerous studies[16–19]. To summarize these, approximately 55% of infarctions were anterior and 45% were inferior. A less favourable outcome was consistently demonstrated for anterior myocardial infarction, with an in-hospital mortality of 15.6% compared with an in-hospital mortality of 9.1% for inferior infarction. This was related not only to the size of the infarction (peak inferior infarction) but also due, in some way, to the location of the infarction (the prognosis remains worse for anterior infarction even when the release of enzymes is similar.)

Strategies in acute myocardial infarction

One of the remaining questions concerning the three major strategies in myocardial infarction is the need for, and the timing of, cardiac catheterization. What spectrum of coronary arterial anatomy will be found if this procedure is performed electively at some time before hospital discharge in patients who have received thrombolysis for acute myocardial infarction? Evidence from the Thrombolysis and Angioplasty in Myocardial Infarction (TAMI) and Thrombolysis in Myocardial Infarction (TIMI) trials suggests that there will be division into the following five angiographic subgroups[20]. The first group, made up of approximately 15% of patients, will have a closed vessel feeding the area of infarction which will not respond to thrombolysis. The second group, again of about 15% of the patients, will have a 'minimal lesion' where occlusive thrombus has presumably formed on a minor plaque, or in the setting of coronary arterial spasm, and lysis has resulted in a widely patent vessel. Follow-up of these patients in the medium term has revealed a relatively high rate of recurrence, but invasive treatment is not required, acutely. The third group, of about 30% of the overall number, will have multivessel disease. The in-hospital course of this group is markedly affected by the anatomy of the vessels not affected by the episode of infarction. The fourth, and largest, group of 35% will have single vessel disease with a greater than, or equal to, 50% residual stenosis. This group has a good prognosis regardless of the degree of stenosis as long as the vessel is patent. The final group, comprising 5% of the patients, will have disease of the main stem of the left coronary artery. These patients will require surgery.

On the basis of these observations, the group from the University of Michigan concluded that the adoption of the 'direct' (primary) strategy of angioplasty results, theoretically at least, in an 'overkill', in which many parients will receive an aggressive treatment which they do not ultimately require, and which may adversely affect their outcome[20].

On the other hand, those advocating the 'direct' approach (no thrombolysis with the patient taken directly to the catheterization laboratory), point to a 25% rate of failure for thrombolysis[7]. They report a significantly improved left ventricular ejection fraction compared with the value prior to angioplasty[21], particularly in those patients with moderate or severe impairment of left ventricular function and cardiogenic shock. There is an improved survival in this latter group, with an overall mortality during the period of hospitalization comparable with that seen with thrombolysis. The shorter, and more predictable, time to reperfusion after mechanical recanalization may contribute to the favourable outcome in experienced centres. Furthermore, the long-term follow-up of the two studies of 'direct' angioplasty that have addressed this issue specifically display impressively low rates of mortality[22,23].

One of the drawbacks in attempting to assess the safety and efficiency of 'direct' angioplasty, none the less, is that there have been no large-scale prospective randomized controlled trials which have compared this approach with intravenous thrombolysis. While comparisons can be made with historical controls, and with recent trials of thrombolysis with or without adjunctive angioplasty, no firm conclusions can be drawn. The largest series of 'direct' angioplasty reported to date is reviewed below.

Direct percutaneous transluminal angioplasty

'Direct' angioplasty was made popular by Hartzler and his colleagues in the early 1980s. It became the standard approach of the Mid America Heart Institute in 1984 for all patients presenting with an acute myocardial infarction. In their experience of 500 patients[23], they report a 94% rate of successful angioplasty and an overall in-hospital mortality of 7.2%. This overall figure is made up of 11.1% for anterior and 5.1% for inferior infarctions. The in-hospital reocclusion rate was 15%. Three aspects of their results deserves special scrutiny:

1. There was a high mortality during the period of hospitalization in patients who underwent failed 'direct' angioplasty (mortality rate 34.3%). This finding has also been reported by other investigators using this approach[22].
2. There was a relatively high in-hospital mortality in patients with multivessel disease (mortality rate 16.1%.
3. A marked improvement in outlook was achieved for those patients with cardiogenic shock (mortality rate 40%).

On follow-up, the rate of restenosis requiring repeat angioplasty was 24%, and a further 13% of the patients underwent late coronary bypass surgery. Of the hospital survivors, 95% were alive at 1 year, and 84% were alive at 5 years. This favourable long-term outcome has also been noted in the smaller series of direct angioplasty.

The 15% rate of reocclusion possibly reflects further trauma to an already 'injured' vessel, in which there is thrombus present. Such rates of reocclusion, however, are not dissimilar to those seen with thrombolysis alone[7,24]. Although it is theoretically possible that the addition of thrombolysis prior to angioplasty could alleviate this problem, experience has not borne this out (see below). The avoidance of thrombolytic agents significantly reduces the incidence of complications due to bleeding[12].

Immediate angioplasty

Carefully designed randomized trials have made major contributions to our understanding of the role of thrombolysis and coronary angioplasty in the short- and long-term management of patients with acute myocardial infarction. The role of the group from the University of Michigan has been central in this respect, and it is from their work that much of the subsequent information is obtained.

If it is assumed that dissolution of fibrin and compression of the plaque is superior to achieving only one or the other of these features then 'immediate' angioplasty is an attractive proposition. In this strategy, thrombolytics are administered as soon as infarction is diagnosed and the patient is transferred immediately to the catheter laboratory for cardiac catheterization, and angioplasty if indicated. Three trials address this question, the TAMI 1[25], the TIMI 2A[26], and the trial of the European Co-operative Study Group (ECSG)[27]. All were prospective and randomized, and all enrolled similar numbers of patients. Although differing slightly in design, all three studies produced comparable results.

All patients received intravenous recombinant tissue-type plasminogen activator and were then randomized to either angioplasty or a deferred strategy which varied according to the trial protocol. Rather against expectations, the combination of thrombolysis followed immediately by angioplasty did not benefit the patient any more than did thrombolysis alone. The more aggressive approach was associated with increased rates of mortality, abrupt closure, reocclusion, need for emergency bypass surgery and complications due to bleeding. No significant difference was found between the left ventricular ejection fractions of patients in either group at the time of their discharge from hospital.

The size of the sample for these trials (there were between 367 and 389 patients in each trial) was calculated on the basis that any difference would be detected in the left ventricular function (the major end-point) between the two groups. The choice of left ventricular function as the major end-point was particularly appropriate since the thrombolytic trials have shown an inconsistent effect on performance of the left ventricle prior to discharge[3,11,28,29], whereas reports from the larger of the direct angioplasty series have generally documented a significant improvement in left ventricular function subsequent to intervention[22,23]. The failure of the trials of 'immediate' angioplasty (thrombolysis followed by angioplasty) to demonstrate this effect may indicate that angioplasty, when linked to thrombolysis in this manner, is not the most appropriate strategy.

One may speculate that mechanical manipulation of a diseased vessel recanalized by thrombolysis inteferes with the process of dissolution of the clot in the diseased segment of that vessel. On the basis of these trials, it seems reasonable to avoid immediate angioplasty if a patient is clinically stable once patency has been achieved by means of thrombolysis following an infarction.

Rescue percutaneous angioplasty

What treatment should be offered to the patient whose vessel feeding the area of infarction has failed to recanalize following thrombolysis? Can this subgroup of patients be shown to derive greater benefit from mechanical intervention following the administration of thrombolytic agents than the previous group? The term 'rescue angioplasty' refers to the strategy of fallback to mechanical recanalization for the treatment of documented failed thrombolysis. Three points should be remembered when reviewing the literature on these patients:

1. As non-responders to medical therapy, they may be relatively resistant to other forms of treatment, and may comprise a group with a poorer prognosis.
2. The time at which a patient is said to have failed thrombolytic therapy is arbitrary (this point was 90 minutes after the administration of thrombolytics in the TAMI trials), and some patients may recanalize late, especially if the non-fibrin specific agents (such as streptokinase or urokinase) have been administered.
3. The use of combinations of agents which are or are not specific for fibrin (for example, recombinant tissue-type plasminogen activator and urokinase) by their differing modes of action, may enhance the overall success of the strategy of rescue angioplasty [30].

Experience with this approach has been variable and the number of patients small. Large randomized controlled trials are required to clarify this issue. A review of four trials revealed a success rate for angioplasty of between 71% and 92%. This is comparable with that seen with 'direct' angioplasty [30–33] but the rate of reocclusion of between 14% and 29% is generally higher than that seen with thrombolysis alone, or with 'direct' angioplasty. It presumably reflects the vigorous thrombogenic forces present in these vessels. The rate of mortality of the two largest trials (10.4% and 17.0%, respectively) are relatively high. The rates of death for those patients who failed both thrombolysis and rescue angioplasty are higher still, and are similar to those seen with failed 'direct' angioplasty. In summary, it seems reasonable to attempt 'rescue' angioplasty in any patients whose clinical condition is unsatisfactory whenever there is thought to be a high likelihood of success.

Angioplasty in cardiogenic shock

These patients represent a special subset whose outlook is exceedingly poor. Their rates of mortality are normally considered to be greater than 80% [34–36]. It will always be an extremely difficult decision whether or not to subject these very ill and unstable patients to a further procedure which they may not even survive, let alone derive benefit. Five series, totalling 98 patients, have been reported [37–41]. These provide grounds for optimism, although no randomized studies have been performed. On pooling the results from there five series, 76% of the patients who underwent successful angioplasty for cardiogenic shock survived, compared with the 24% who survived when angioplasty was unsuccessful. This result can be compared with the overall pooled survival rate from the four surgical series in which emergency coronary arterial bypass surgery was performed for cardiogenic shock. Of these patients, 72% survived [42–45].

Therefore, a very aggressive policy for this condition will almost certainly save lives. More information is required, however, before this stance can be recommended. At this stage, the procedure must be reserved for those patients fulfilling universally agreed clinical criteria.

Protected angioplasty

Protected angioplasty may enhance the safety and effectiveness of intervention during acute myocardial infarction. The term 'protection' covers any intervention designed to reduce myocardial ischaemia, and can be broadly classified into pharmacological and mechanical methods. Only the latter approach will be described here, apart from noting that pretreatment with intravenous lignocaine, intracoronary nitrates, calcium antagonists or beta blockers has been reported to allow safer and more prolonged inflations of balloon catheters[46–48].

There are several techniques under investigation. Although they have not yet been specifically applied to the patient undergoing angiography in the context of acute infarction, there are obvious clinical implications for their use in this situation.

The bailout catheter and perfusion balloon catheter have been designed to assist in the management of acute closure complicating elective angioplasty[49]. These catheters have side-holes located proximal in the shaft and distal to the segment supporting the balloon, along with a central lumen that permits the passage of a pulsatile flow of blood. At mean systemic arterial pressures of 80 mm Hg, between 40 and 60 ml of blood per minute can be transmitted via this lumen. The perfusion balloon catheter has the additional capacity of dilatation of stenoses. The rationale for its use is that longer inflations (15–30 minutes) may reduce subsequent rates of restenosis by inducing local intimal, and medial, ischaemia. Long inflations at low pressure in the event of acute closure may also be more effective at 'tacking down' the intimal flap[50,51].

The role of these catheters in acute myocardial infarction remains to be evaluated. The presence of extensive thrombus, as is sometimes seen in this setting, may block the side-holes, despite adequate anticoagulation and thrombolysis. These devices have a relatively high profile and positioning the device correctly in the vessel feeding the area of infarction may be time consuming, difficult, or even impossible. In addition, the systemic blood pressure must be stable to provide an adequate driving pressure.

Myocardial perfusion devices

There are several of these devices available[52,53]. They function in a similar way as those already described, except that coronary arterial perfusion is active rather than passive. Blood or oxygenated fluorocarbon compounds (Fluosol DA 20%) are used. Oxygenated blood is taken from either a renal vein (in which the saturations of oxygen are between 85 and 92% despite passage through the kidney) or from the femoral artery. The blood is then pumped via a catheter into the coronary artery distal to the obstruction (antegrade flow), or pumped via a specially designed catheter into the coronary sinus to provide retrograde perfusion[54,55]. Retroperfusion is synchronized to diastole to allow normal venous drainage to occur in systole. The major limitation of these techniques is in maintaining an adequate flow of blood through small-gauge catheters without inducing significant haemolysis.

Mechanical unloading of the left ventricle

The intra-aortic balloon pump and the haemopump may be used to stabilize the patient during emergency angioplasty. Intra-aortic balloon counterpulsation has been used historically in the treatment of patients with cardiogenic shock to improve perfusion of tissues and reduce the extent of infarction, and also in those patients with the syndrome of unstable angina[56]. Despite the clinical improvement seen in shocked patients, the evidence for reduction of the extent of infarction and improvement in rate of mortality is unconvincing[57]. Haemodynamic studies show that the cardiac output is increased by up to 20% with lower systolic and diastolic pressures. Coronary flow is also improved, but to a lesser extent[58]. The value of intra-aortic balloon counterpulsation during angioplasty for acute myocardial infarction has not been specifically addressed in trials, but it is generally considered useful in the unstable patient.

The haemopump is a circulatory assist device consisting of a motor-driven turbine located within a 21F catheter. The device is positioned via the femoral artery so that its tip is located within the left ventricle. Blood is then sucked from the left ventricle and liberated in the descending aorta[59]. A cardiac output of between 3 litres/min and 4 litres/min can be achieved. The advantages of this device include the peripheral approach (and this will probably be by percutaneous puncture after miniaturization of the device) and almost total decompression of the left ventricule with a marked reduction in demand for myocardial oxygen. It has the ability to function as a bridge to transplantation should this be required. Patients with extensive areas of stunned myocardium may be expected to derive the greatest benefit. Its disadvantages include the potential for haemolysis or thrombosis, and injury to the peripheral arterial vasculature[20].

Percutaneous cardiopulmonary support

Those patients judged to be at high risk of haemodynamic collapse, either during prolonged inflation of balloons or after acute closure of vessels, or who are unstable as a result of their acute myocardial infarction, may be stabilized by percutaneous cardiopulmonary support[60,61]. Access to the vasculature is via the femoral vein and artery. The procedure is performed under local anaesthetic. With an output from the pump of 4–6 litres/min, the arterial pressure can be maintained at 70–80 mm Hg with a pulse pressure of 10 mm Hg (the small pulse pressure presumably reflecting the contribution from the patient). This results in satisfactory perfusion with good mentation and adequate output of urine even at times of cardiac arrest. Full anticoagulation is required, and this is not reversed at the end of the procedure since the administration of protamine has been associated with acute closure of vessels.

This technique not only assists the operator performing an angioplasty, but also facilitates transfer to surgery if required, and provides a satisfactory haemodynamic state in which the internal mammary artery may be utilized by the surgeon.

Conclusion

Thrombolysis is now firmly established in the treatment of acute myocardial infarction. The precise role of angioplasty is not so clear. The larger trials of 'direct' angioplasty (angioplasty without thrombolysis) strongly suggest that this treatment can be performed in experienced centres with a high level of success. The rates of mortality during the stay in hospital compare favourably with thrombolysis, and the rates of death from 1 to 3 year follow-up appear superior. No prospective randomized controlled trials have been carried out, however, and these are required before definite recommendations can be made. The considerable logistical back-up required for such a strategy means that it is unlikely to become extensively available. The optimal treatment of those patients who fail to respond to thrombolysis remains unclear, but decisions should be made on the basis of the clinical situation and the coronary arterial anatomy. It seems clear that those patients who remain unstable, and who have severe multivessel disease, are better treated by complete revascularization. Reliable non-invasive methods (such as assessment of late potentials) are required to determine the patency of the arteries. Finally, the outlook for cardiogenic shock may improve with the adoption of a more aggressive approach but randomized trials of emergency angioplasty and possibly emergency surgery are required.

Acknowledgement

We are indebted to the secretarial assistance of Ruth Easton during the preparation of the manuscript.

References

1. Gruppo Italiano per lo Studio della Streptochinasi nell 'Infarto Miocardio (GISSI). Effectiveness of intravenous thrombolytic treatment in acute myocardial infarction. *Lancet*, **i**, 397–401, 1986
2. ISIS-2 (Second International Study of Infarct Survival) Collaborative Group. Randomised trial of intravenous streptokinase, oral aspirin, both, or neither among 17 187 cases of suspected acute myocardial infarction: ISIS-2. *Lancet*, **ii**, 349–360, 1988
3. The ISAM Study Group. A prospective trial of intravenous streptokinase in acute myocardial infarction (ISAM). *N. Engl. J. Med.*, **314**, 1465–1471, 1986
4. Wilcox, R.G., von der Lppe, G., Olsson, C.G., *et al.* Trial of tissue plasminogen activator for mortality reduction in active myocardial infarction. *Lancet*, **ii**, 525–530, 1988
5. The TIMI Study Group. The thrombolysis in myocardial infarction (TIMI) trial. *N. Engl. J. Med.*, **312**, 932–936, 1985
6. Hills, L.D., Borer, J., Braunwald, E., *et al.* High dose intravenous streptokinase for acute myocardial infarction: Preliminary results of a multicenter trial. *J. Am. Coll. Cardiol.*, **6**, 957–962, 1985
7. O'Niell, W., Timmis, G.C., Bourdillon, P.D., *et al.* A prospective randomised clinical trial of intracoronary streptokinase VS coronary angioplasty for acute myocardial infarction. *N. Engl. J. Med.*, **314**, 812–818, 1986
8. PRIMI Trial Study Group. Randomised double-blind trial of recombinant prourokinase against streptokinase in acute myocardial infarction. *Lancet*, **ii**, 863–868, 1989
9. Yusuf, S., Collins, R., Peto, R., *et al.* Intravenous and intracoronary fibrinolytic therapy in acute myocardial infarction: Overview of results on mortality, reinfarction and side effects from 33 randomised controlled trials. *Eur. Heart J.*, **6**, 556–585, 1985
10. Kennedy, J.W., Martin, G.V., Davis, K.B., *et al.* The western Washington Intravenous Streptokinase in Acute Myocardial Infarction randomised trial. *Circulation*, **77**, 345–352, 1988
11. White, H.D., Norris, R.M., Brown, M.A., *et al.* Effect of intravenous streptokinase on left ventricular function and early survival after acute myocardial infarction. *N. Engl. J. Med.*, **317**, 850–855, 1987
12. Cairns, J.A., Collins, R., Fuster, V. and Passamani, E.R. Coronary thrombolysis. *Chest*, **95**, 73S–87S, 1989
13. Thorsen, L.I., Brosstad, F., Gogstad, *et al.* Competitions between fibrinogen with its degradation products for interactions with the platelet-fibrinogen receptor. *Thromb. Res.*, **44**, 611–623, 1986
14. Mark, D.B., Hlatky, M.A., O'Connor, C.M., *et al.* Administration of thrombolytic therapy in the community hospital: Established principles and unresolved issues. *J. Am. Coll. Cardiol.*, **12**, 32A–43A, 1988
15. De Wood, M.A., Spores, J., Notske, R., *et al.* Prevalence of total coronary occlusion during the early hours of transmural myocardial infarction. *N. Engl. J. Med.*, **303**, 897–902, 1980

16. Stadius, M.L., Davis, K., Maynard, C., *et al.* Risk stratification for one year survival based on characteristics identified in the eary hours of myocardial infarction. *Circulation,* **74,** 703–711, 1986

17. Roubin, G.S., Harris, P.J., Bernstein, L. and Kelly, D.T. Coronary anatomy and prognosis after myocardial infarction in parients 60 years and younger. *Circulation,* **67,** 743–749, 1983

18. Sanz, G., Castaner, A., Betrice, A., *et al.* Determinants of prognosis in survivors of myocardial infarction. *N. Engl. J. Med.,* **306,** 1065–1070, 1982

19. Taylor, G.J., Humphries, J.O., Mellits, E.D., *et al.* Predictors of clinical course, coronary anatomy and left ventricular function after recovery from acute myocardial infarction. *Circulation,* **62,** 960–970, 1980

20. Topol, E.J. Mechanical Interventions for Acute Myocardial Infarction. In *Textbook of Interventional Cardiology* (ed. E.J. Topol), Saunders, Philadelphia, pp. 269–299, 1990

21. Stone, G.W., Rutherford, B.D., McLonahay, D.R., *et al.* Direct coronary angioplasty in acute myocardial infarction: Outcome in patients with single vessel disease. *J. Am. Coll. Cardiol.,* **15,** 534–543, 1990

22. Rothburn, D.A., Linnermeir, R.J., Landin, E.J., *et al.* Emergency percutaneous transluminal coronary angioplasty in acute myocardial infarction: a three year experience. *J. Am. Coll. Cardiol.,* **10,** 264–272, 1987

23. O'Keefe, J.H., Jr., Rutherford, B.D., McLonahay, D.R., *et al.* Early and late results of coronary angioplasty without antecedent thrombolytic therapy for acute myocardial infarction. *Am. J, Cardiol.,* **64,** 1221–1230, 1989

24. Erbel, R., Pop, T., Dufenbach, C. and Meyer, J. Longterm results of thrombolytic therapy with and without percutaneous transluminal coronary angioplasty. *J. Am. Coll. Cardiol.,* **14,** 276–285, 1989

25. Topol, E.J., Califf, R.M., George, B.S., *et al.* A randomised trial of immediate versus delayed elective angioplasty after intravenous tissue plasminogen activator in acute mycoardial infarction. *N. Engl. J. Med.,* **317,** 581–588, 1987

26. TIMI Research Group. Immediate Vs delayed catheterisation and angioplasty following thrombolytic therapy for acute myocardial infarction. *J. Am. Med. Assoc.,* **260,** 2849–2858, 1988

27. Simoons, M.L., Arnold, A.E.R., Bower, R.W., *et al.* Thrombolysis with rt-PA in acute myocardial infarction: no beneficial effects of immediate PTCA. *Lancet,* **i,** 197–203, 1988

28. Kennedy, J.W., Martin, G.V., Davis, K.B., *et al.* The Western Washington intravenous streptokinase in acute myocardial infarction randomised trial. *Circulation,* **77,** 345–352, 1988

29. Van de Werf, F. and Arnold, A.E.R. Intravenous tissue plasminogen activator and size of infarct, left ventricular function and survival in acute myocardial infarction. *Br. Med. J.,* **297,** 1373–1379, 1988

30. Topol, E.J., Califf, R.M., George, B.S., *et al.* Coronary arterial thrombolysis with combined infusion of recombinant tissue-type plasminogen activator and urokinase in patients with acute myocardial infarction. *Circulation,* **77,** 1100–1107, 1988

31. Califf, R.M., Topol, E.J. and George, B.S. Characteristics and outcome of patients in whom reperfusion with intravenous tissue-type plasminogen activator fails. Results of the thrombolysis and angioplasty in Myocardial Infarction (TAMI) 1 trial. *Circulation,* **77,** 1090–1099, 1988

32. O'Connor, C.M., Mark, D.B., Hinohara, T., *et al.* Rescue coronary angioplasty after failure of intravenous streptokinase in acute myocardial infarction. In-hospital and long term outcomes. *J. Invest. Cardiol.,* **1,** 85–95, 1989

33. Baim, D.S., Diver, D.J., Knatterud, G.L. and the TIMI II A Investigators. PTCA 'salvage' for thrombolytic failures – implications from TIMI II A. *Circulation,* **78 (Suppl. 11),** 11–112, 1988

34. Loeb, H.S., Rahimtoola, S.H. and Gunnar, R.M. The failing myocardium: 1 Drug management. *Med. Clin. North Am.,* **57,** 167–185, 1974

35. Da Luz, P., Weil, H. and Shubin, H. Current concepts on mechanisms and treatment of cardiogenic shock. *Am. Heart J.,* **92,** 103–113, 1976

36. Scheidt, S., Wilner, G., Mueller, H., *et al.* Intraaortic balloon counterpulsation in cardiogenic shock: Report of a cooperative clinical trial. *N. Engl. J. Med.,* **288,** 979–984, 1973

37. O'Neill, W., Erbel, R., Laufer, N., *et al.* Coronary angioplasty therapy of cardiogenic shock complicating acute myocardial infarction. *Circulation,* **72,** III–309, 1985

38. Lee, L., Bates, E.R., Pitt, B., *et al.* Percutaneous transluminal coronary angioplasty improves survival in acute myocardial infarction complicated by cardiogenic shock. *Circulation,* **78,** 1345–1351, 1988

39. Shani, J., Rivera, M., Greengart, A., *et al.* Percutaneous transluminal coronary angioplasty in cardiogenic shock. *J. Am. Coll. Cardiol.,* **7,** 149A, 1986

40. Heuser, R.R., Maddoux, G.L., Goss, F.E., *et al.* Coronary angioplasty for acute mitral regurgitation due to myocardial infarction. *Ann. Int. Med.,* **107,** 852–855, 1987

41. Brown, T.M., Jr., Iannone, L.A., Gordon, D.F., *et al.* Percutaneous myocardial perfusion (PMR) reduces mortality in acute myocardial infarction (MI) complicated by cardiogenic shock. *Circulation,* **72,** III–309, 1985

42. De Wood, M.A., Notske, R.N., Hensley, G.R., *et al.* Intraaortic balloon counterpulsations with and without reperfusion for myocardial infarction shock. *Circulation*, **61**, 1105–1112, 1980
43. Phillips, S.J., Zeff, R.H., Skinner, J.R., *et al.* Reperfusion protocol and results in 738 patients with evolving myocardial infarction. *Ann. Thorac. Surg.*, **41**, 119–125, 1986
44. Guyton, R.A., Arcidi, J.M., Jr., Langford, D.A., *et al.* Emergency coronary bypass for cardiogenic shock. *Circulation*, **76(Suppl. V)**, V-22, 1987
45. Laks, H., Rosenbranz, E. and Buckberg, G.D. Surgical treatments of cardiogenic shock after myocardial infarction. *Circulation*, **74(Suppl. III)**, 111–115, 1986
46. Erbel, R., Schreiner, G., Henkel, B., *et al.* Improved ischaemic tolerance following transluminal coronary angioplasty by intracoronary injection of nitroglycerin. *Z. Kardiol.*, **72(Suppl. III)**, 71–73, 1983
47. Schreiner, G., Erbel, R., Henkel, B., *et al.* Improved ischaemic tolerance during percutaneous transluminal coronary angioplasty (PTCA) by antianginal drugs (abstract). *Circulation*, **00 (Suppl. 111)**, 111–198, 1983
48. Zalewski, A., Goldberg, S.D., Dervan, J.P., *et al.* Myocardial protection during transient coronary artery occlusion in man. Beneficial effects or regional beta-adrenergic blockade. *Circulation*, **73**, 734–739, 1986
49. Kereiakes, D.J. and Stack, R.S. Perfusion angioplasty. In *Textbook of International Cardiology* (ed. E.J. Topol), Saunders, Philadelphia, pp. 452–465, 1990
50. Perez, J.A., Milkat, E.M., Ramires, N.M., *et al.* Effect of prolonged balloon inflation on arterial hyperplasia in rabbits (abstract). *Circulation*, **76 (Suppl. IV)**, IV–184, 1987
51. Stack, R.S., Quigley, P.J., Collins, G. and Phillips, H.R. Perfusion balloon catheter. *Am. J. Cardiol.*, **61**, 779–809, 1988
52. Lehmann, K.G., Atwood, J.E., Synder, E.L. and Ellison, R.L. Autologous blood perfusion for myocardial protection during coronary angioplasty. A feasibility study. *Circulation*, **76**, 312–323, 1987
53. Clemon, M., Jaffee, U. and Wholgelernter, D. Prevention of ischaemia during percutaneous transluminal coronary angioplasty by catheter infusion of oxygenated Fluosol DA 20%. *Circulation*, **74**, 555–562, 1986
54. Kas, S., Drury, J.K., Eigler, N., *et al.* Coronary venous retroperfusion reduces ischaemia during LAD angioplasty. *Circulation*, **78**, II–104, 1988
55. Berland, J., Farcot, J.C., Barrier, A., *et al.* ECG and 2D echo assessment of myocardial protection achieved by diastolic synchronised coronary sinus retroperfusion (DSR) during LAD angioplasty. *J. Am. Coll. Cardiol.*, **11**, 132A, 1988
56. Bolooki, H. *Clinical Application of Intra-aortic Balloon Pump*, Future Publishing, Mt Kisco, NY, 1977.
57. Williams, D.O., Korr, K.S., Gerwirtz, H. and Most, A.S. The effect of intra-aortic balloon conterpulsation on regional myocardial blood flow and oxygen consumption in the presence of coronary artery stenosis in patients with unstable angina. *Circulation*, **66**, 593–597, 1982
58. O'Rouke, M.F., Norse, R.M., Campbell, T.J., *et al.* Randomised controlled trial of intra-aortic balloon counterpulsation in early myocardial infarction with acute heart failure. *Am. J. Cardiol.*, **47**, 815, 1981
59. Frazier, O.H., Wampler, R.K., Duncan, J.M., *et al.* First human use of haemopump, a catheter-mounted ventricular assist device. *J. Am. Coll. Cardiol.*, **13**, 121A, 1989
60. Vogel, R.A., Tommaso, C. and Gundry, S. Initial experience with an angioplasty and aortic valvuloplasty using elective semipercutaneous cardiopulmonary support. *Am. J. Cardiol.*, **62**, 811–813, 1988
61. Vogel, R.A. The Maryland Experience: Angioplasty and valvuloplasty using percutaneous cardiopulmonary support. *Am. J. Cardiol.*, **62**, 11k.–14k., 1988

10

Coronary arterial endothelium in ischaemia

Peter Collins

Introduction

In the last 20 years, it has been discovered that the vascular endothelium which lines the entire circulatory system is not merely a passive diffusion barrier. Instead, it represents a fully functional organ with a variety of biological functions. It is an anti-thrombogenic surface, and regulates both coagulation and fibrinolysis. It is able to synthesize and release heparan sulphate[1], antithrombin III[2], prostacyclin[3], and plasminogen activator[4]. These substances maintain the fluidity of the blood at the interface between it and the vessel wall, and prevent adherence of both red cells and platelets. Other substances, such as von Willebrand factor[5], fibronectin[6], and thrombospondin[7], are synthesized by the endothelium and are involved in formation of localized thrombus. Other important functions of the endothelium include the metabolism of noradrenaline[8], serotonin[9] and adenine nucleo-tides[10]. It contains angiotensin converting enzyme[11] and other peptidases. In 1980, however, Furchgott and Zawadzki[12] discovered that the endothelium itself could have a potent relaxing effect on the smooth muscle of the vascular wall. Studies on isolated arterial preparations, including coronary arteries, demonstrated an obligatory role for endothelial cells in the dilatory responses of vascular smooth muscle to various neurohumoral agents. This phenomenon is due to so-called endothelium-derived relaxing factor. Removal of the endothelium abolishes the dilatation observed in response to treatment with acetylcholine, bradykinin, throm-bin and substance P[13,14], and potentiates the vasoconstrictor responses to serotonin[15] (Figure 10.1).

The modulation of vascular tone mediated by the relaxing factor has been demonstrated in many large conductance arteries like the coronary arteries and aorta[16,12]. In such vessels, however, vasomotion does not determine the rate of tissue perfusion unless critical narrowings are present. The role of vasomotion mediated by the relaxing factor in resistance vessels, which are responsible for control of perfusion of the tissues, has not yet been well established. This is because there have been difficulties in functionally inhibiting, or destroying, the endothelium in a defined manner without causing simultaneous damage to the adjacent tissue. Evidence is accumulating, none the less, that vasomotion mediated by the endothe-lium plays a significant role in the micro-circulation of various beds.

Physicochemical release of endothelium-derived relaxing factor in coronary arteries

Substances shown to cause endothelium-dependent dilatation

Peptides have endothelium-dependent vasodilator effects; substance P[19] and calcitonin gene-related peptide[20,21] are potent dilators of human epicardial coronary arteries and their dilatory effects are endothelium dependent in preparations studied *in vitro*. These peptides have the advantage that they are pure vasodilators, with no direct constricting effect on smooth muscle, this latter action being the disadvantage of acetylcholine. Another peptide, vasoactive intestinal polypeptide, has been shown to relax the bovine intrapulmonary artery by an endothelium-dependent mechanism[22]. Evidence for an endothelium-dependent relaxation response to acetylcholine in the human coronary artery has been conflicting. In one study[23], using rings of human coronary arteries studied *in vitro*, it proved difficult to demonstrate acetylcholine-induced dilatation in the presence of endothelium. When human epicardial artery rings were obtained from the hearts of transplant recipients or donors, free from serious atherosclerosis, acetylcholine was shown to have a relaxing effect. In a more recent study[24], using quantitative angiography, acetylcholine was shown to cause a dose-dependent dilatation in normal coronary arteries. This effect was lost in coronary arteries with advanced atheromatous disease. These findings suggest that an abnormal vascular response to acetylcholine may represent a defect in endothelial vasodilator function which may be important in the pathogenesis of coronary vasospasm[24]. This specificity of an effective response to acetylcholine in the human coronary arteries lacking endothelium, and the acetylcholine response itself, is conflicting.

There have been no studies that have investigated the specific effect of acetylcholine response on the velocity of flow of blood in the coronary arteries and the vasodilatory reserve in man. The specificity of any relaxing effect from the endothelium has not been tested with known inhibitors of the relaxing factor. A large number of the inhibitors of the relaxing factor derived from the endothelium would be totally unsuitable for clinical use, since many of them are powerful anti-oxidants and these would be highly toxic in man. Activity derived from the endothelium, however, could possibly be assessed by using a safe but specific inhibitor. Such an inhibitor is haemoglobin[25,26]. Free haemoglobin has been used as a blood substitute in the past and, at the local doses needed to inhibit the relaxing factor (10^{-5} mol-l), would be safe[27,28]. The relaxing factor itself has recently been shown to be nitric oxide[29] or a substance containing nitric oxide such as S-nitrosocysteine[30]. Haemoglobin inhibits its action by combining directly with the nitric oxide molecule[29]. Haemoglobin has also been shown to inhibit activity of the factor induced by increased flow[31], and does not increase vascular tone in the absence of endothelium[26,32,33]. It should thus be possible, specifically, to block any vasodilatory effect of the factor derived from endothelium by using haemoglobin. Also, because the factor is an autocoid, inhibition by haemoglobin will be acute, with no possibility of longer term effects, since once the complex between haemoglobin and nitric oxide is formed and is cleared, no further inhibition would be anticipated.

As well as its potent relaxing effect on vascular smooth muscle, the factor derived from the endothelium has been reported to inhibit aggregation of platelets[34,35]. In this respect, it inhibits thrombin-stimulated adhesion of platelets to mono layers of bovine endothelial cells[36]. There is only one report to show that it influences

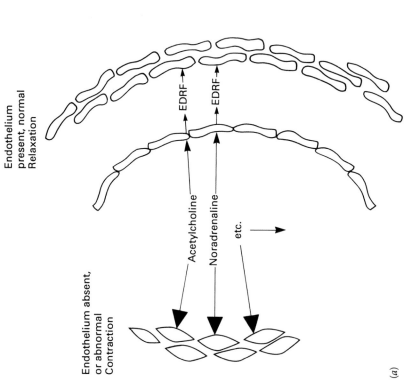

(a)

Figure 10.1 (a) Various physicochemical agents can cause vessel relaxation in the presence of endothelium via a release of endothelium-derived relaxing factor (right-hand side). Conversely, in the absence of endothelium, these agents will result in constriction of the vessel (left-hand side). (b) Endothelial cells have receptors to various agents on their surface: muscarinic receptor (M), alpha₂ receptor (α₂), P receptor, thrombin receptor. This will result in the release of a factor derived from the endothelium and relaxation of the smooth muscle. Smooth muscle cells also have these receptors on their surface, and direct activation of the latter receptors will result in contraction

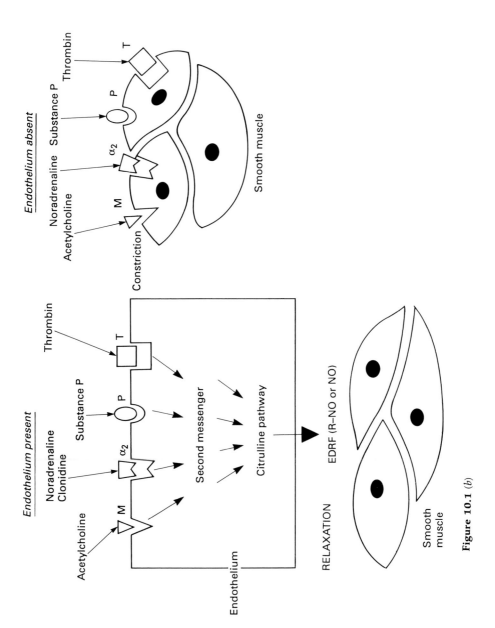

Figure 10.1 (*b*)

function of platelets *in vivo* [37]. This study was performed in the rabbit, and showed that release of the factor inhibited aggregation of platelets and elevation of content of cyclic-GMP within platelets. These effects were reversed by the inhibition with haemoglobin.

Flow-mediated endothelium-dependent dilatation

Another important, and recent, finding is that there is a flow-mediated, endothelium-dependent dilatation of epicardial coronary arteries in the conscious dog [17]. This flow-dependent dilatation has been shown to be due to an increase in release of the endothelial-derived relaxing factor [18], brought about by the increase in rate of flow, detected by an increase in shear stress on the endothelial cell wall which, in turn, causes a release of the factor (Figure 10.2).

Disease states

Atherosclerosis

Endothelium-dependent relaxation is impaired in arteries obtained from atherosclerotic rabbits [38], monkeys [39] and man [40]. Attempts to quantify the release of the relaxing factor from the endothelium of atheromatous arteries have produced conflicting results. In a rabbit preparation, one group found no reduction in release of

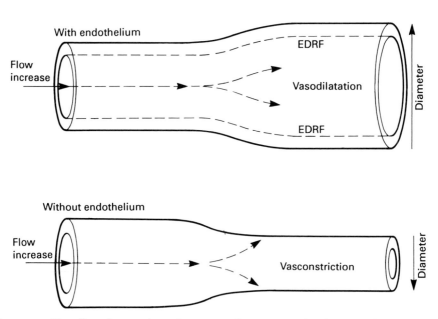

Figure 10.2 The effect of an *intraluminal* increase in flow in a vessel with (top) and one without (bottom) endothelium. An increase in flow in the vessel with its endothelial lining causes an increase in its diameter. Conversely, in the absence of endothelium, increased flow produces a decrease in diameter

the factor in the lumen[41], while another group found a reduced release[42]. In monkeys, this impairment is not due to a generalized defect in endothelium caused by hypocholesterolaemia, but requires the presence of atherosclerosis[39]. Furthermore, the impairment of endothelium-dependent relaxation caused by feeding rabbits diets rich in cholesterol could be reduced by low doses of a dihydropyridine calcium antagonist[43]. Another recent study in monkeys shows a restoration of endothelium-dependent relaxation by dietary treatment of atherosclerosis[44]. The intima remained thickened after regression of the atherosclerosis which suggests that this does not prevent the factor, derived from the endothelium, from reaching the underlying vascular smooth muscle.

Atheroma impairs the endothelium-dependent relaxation in large isolated and atherosclerotic coronary arteries from humans[40]. It has also been demonstrated that, in patients with coronary arterial disease, acetylcholine causes a dose-dependent constriction of any diseased arterial segments compared with a dose-dependent dilatation in normal coronary arteries[24]. Nitroglycerine, however, produced dilatation in both atheromatous and normal coronary arteries. This would imply a loss of normal endothelial vasodilator function in coronary arterial disease. These findings, in both experimental and human atheroma, would suggest there is an increase in response of smooth muscle to constrictor agents in the vicinity of atheromatous lesions, possibly due to reduced activity of the factor derived from the endothelium (Figure 10.3). Such constriction could well change a non-critical stenosis of a coronary artery into a critical one, with consequent myocardial ischaemia. A beneficial effect of dietary supplementation with cod-liver oil has been shown in endothelium-dependent responses in porcine coronary arteries[45]. These data suggest that the cod-liver oil facilitates endothelium-dependent relaxation in the tissue.

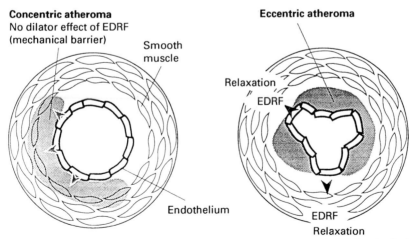

Figure 10.3 The effect of atheroma on endothelium-dependent relaxation. The left-hand side shows concentric atheroma resulting in a mechanical barrier between the released relaxation factor and the underlying smooth muscle. The right-hand side shows the effect of eccentric atheroma. At sites of atheroma there will be a mechanical barrier between the factor released, but there are areas without atheroma where the factor will be able to penetrate the smooth muscle. Such sites will relax, and overall there may be sufficient effect from the endothelially derived factor to allow net relaxation of the vessel

Hypertension

The relaxant effects of endothelium-dependent (acetylcholine–histamine) and endothelium-dependent (nitroprusside, nitrite) relaxing substances were examined on rings from the thoracic aorta of normotensive and experimentally hypertensive rats[46]. It was found that, in preparations from the hypertensive animals, there was a highly significant depression of the endothelium-dependent relaxation brought about by histamine and acetylcholine. This was not seen with nitroprusside and nitrate. There was no decrease in release of relaxing factor, and it was thought that the impaired coupling between endothelium and smooth muscle cells accounted for the differences. This may have been due to the fact that, in hypertensive rats, there was marked thickening of the sub-endothelial cells which could increase the distance between the endothelial cell layer and the total mass of smooth muscle cells[47].

In another study in dogs, acute coronary hypertension caused endothelial damage and potentiated the constrictor response to serotonin in the coronary artery[48]. Coarctation-induced hypertension in rabbits was associated with diminished relaxation by endothelium-dependent agonists[49]. The endothelium-dependent relaxation was only impaired above the coarctation. Endothelium-dependent relaxation to nitroprusside was not impaired, suggesting that this inhibition of such relaxation is due to a local response to the elevation of blood pressure, and not due to a circulating factor. This effect may account for some of the pathological states that occur in hypertension, such as decrease in the reserve for coronary flow and atheroma.

Is endothelium-derived nitric oxide important in human coronary arteries?

Recently, we have investigated the possible involvement of a factor derived from endothelium in the control of coronary arterial diameter and flow in human subjects with normal coronary arteries. Preliminary results suggest that endothelium-derived nitric oxide is an important factor in the control of the diameters of human coronary arteries during life.

Acetylcholine causes a dose-dependent dilatation in normal coronary arteries. This effect is lost in advanced coronary atheromatous disease, suggesting that an abnormal vascular response to acetylcholine may represent a defect in endothelial vasodilator function. This may be important in the pathogenesis of coronary vasospasm. It has also recently been reported that N^G monomethyl-$=$-arginine (L-NMMA), a specific inhibitor of the synthesis of endothelium-derived nitric oxide, inhibits the basal flow of blood and attenuates the dilator response to infused acetylcholine, but not glyceryltrinitrate in the brachial arteries of healthy volunteers[50].

Potential clinical significance of altered composition of the vessel wall

It is well known that infiltration with cells is a common finding in the vessel wall around developing atheroma. Chemical mediators of inflammation, released from infiltrating leucocytes, may play a key role in the hyper-responsiveness of epicardial coronary arteries in patients with vasospastic angina. There are data to support this hypothesis, suggesting an imbalance in the local interaction of endothelial cells, smooth muscle cells, and inflammatory cells as a pathophysiological mechanism of coronary spasm.

It has been observed clinically that patients with developing coronary arterial disease have a period of more 'vasotonic' angina, which may precede fixed obstructive disease[50]. There appears to be a typical waxing and waning period of symptoms due to the dynamic aspect of the coronary arterial obstructions.

Infiltration of mast cells around atheroma in coronary arteries is well known[51]. Activated mast cells are known to release several inflammatory mediators and substances which have a high constrictive potency. Some patients have been described who have died from coronary spasm, with a sudden cardiac death, but there is a substantial accumulation of mast cells in the atherosclerotic coronary artery at the site of the previously angiographically documented spasm[52]. Some of the identified mediators are potent constrictors, such as histamine, serotonin, leuko-trienes C4 and D4, and prostaglandin D2. Many of these agents, in the presence of endothelium, are, however, vasodilators and, therefore, the constriction may be counteracted in the presence of endothelium. Probably the provocation of coronary spasm by histamine of the 5-hydroxytryptamine receptor agonist ergonovine can be explained by the loss of endothelial protection, either due to localized damage or metabolic dysfunction at this site.

A typical feature of vasospastic angina is circadian periodicity of the attacks. Interestingly, there is a circadian periodicity of plasma free-fatty acids concentra-tion[53], which may affect endothelial function such as LDL-receptor endocyto-sis[54]. The important question is whether this relates to intramural or mast cell activation and, as yet, this question has not been answered. Thus, an altered cellular composition of the coronary arterial wall, due to inflammation in response to developing atheromatous disease, could result in constrictive hyper-reactivity of the wall. Endothelial dilators may modify the reactivity of the artery to constrictive mediators released from mast cells. Indeed, this has been shown in man for aggregating platelets, where endothelium modifies the aggregability of platelets taken from animals in which the endothelium has been damaged[55].

Clinical implications

Unstable angina

It could be hypothesized that the loss of endothelium-mediated vasodilatation may contribute to vascular hyper-reactivity to various conditions and pharmacological substances (Figure 10.4). As has already been mentioned, atherosclerotic arteries appear to have a reduced endothelium-mediated vasomotion[38,39]. Interestingly, hypercholesterolaemia alone has been shown to reduce acetylcholine-induced, endothelium-dependent dilatation[56]. A large number of compounds acting as endothelium-dependent dilators will cause constriction when they have direct access to the smooth muscle without the protection of the endothelium-mediated vasomo-tor effect. A re-growth in turnover process during endothelial repair may explain the pronounced vascular instability repeatedly observed in conditions following endoth-elial damage and impairment[57]. This process may also be involved in the rapidly changing threshold levels often observed in effort angina[57,58]. These endothelium-dependent mechanisms may contribute to the sudden change in the pattern of symptoms which occurs in unstable angina. A better understanding of endothelial function in this condition may lead to new approaches for its prevention and its treatment.

Myocardial infarction

There is now a wealth of literature to suggest that acute myocardial infarction, and sudden death, is frequently associated with freshly ruptured plaque[59,60], sometimes with relatively little formation of thrombus[61]. The sudden exposure of collagen fibres, activating platelets and the release of their vasoactive material, plus a sudden loss of local endothelium-mediated vasodilator influence, may result in excessive local vasoconstriction. A release of products of platelet, such as 5-hydroxytryptamine, thrombin, adenosine triphosphate and adenosine diphosphate, will not be able to elicit dilatation via endothelium during this condition, but will directly stimulate smooth muscle and cause local hyper-responsiveness. Of course, the intima itself may be damaged by the resulting ischaemia, further impairing endothelium-mediated dilatation[62]. This may also occur in areas directly adjacent to the zone of ischaemia, resulting in a positive feedback mechanism which causes increased platelet activation and release of vasoactive substances. This, then, further compounds the endothelium-mediated dilatation and prejudices vasomotor homeostasis. Coronary arterial constriction may then lead to arterial occlusion or myocardial infarction. Some of this is speculation at the moment, but there is intense research

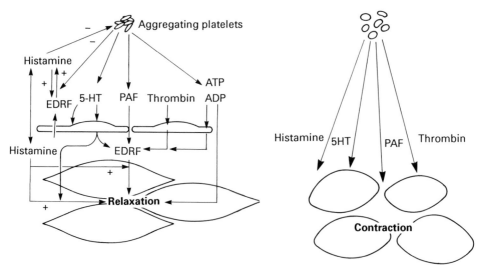

Figure 10.4 This diagram demonstrates how an intact endothelium can 'protect' the vessel from vasoconstrictive substances released from aggregating platelets. In the absence of endothelium (right-hand side), platelets aggregate on the surface of the smooth muscle with the release of constricting agents such has histamine, 5-hydroxy tryptamine and thrombin. Constriction of smooth muscle will occur. In the presence of endothelium, these platelet-derived agents will cause the release of an endothelially derived relaxant factor abluminally and luminally which will result in the relaxation of smooth muscle and inhibition of further aggregation of platelets

going on in this field which will, hopefully, improve our understanding and treatment of this condition.

Angioplasty-induced endothelial damage

Localized coronary spasm after successful coronary angioplasty has been observed after the treatment of significant coronary arterial stenoses[63,64]. While there is compression and damage to the intima, fissures and dissections occur[63]. Exposure of the smooth muscle directly leads to local release of circulating vasomotor compounds, which, in the absence of a protective endothelium may contribute to enhanced vasoconstriction. During the healing process, the formation of a functioning endothelium causes a progressive disappearance of this excessive tendency towards vasoconstriction. The alteration in vascular tone is quite distinct from the organic phenomenon of restenosis, which is seen within 3–6 months after an angioplasty and is frequently observed in approximately one-third of all patients[65]. It would appear that a regrowth of endothelium over the site of angioplasty is one of the determinants of restenosis. There are some reports that nitric oxide may have the ability to inhibit the proliferation of vascular smooth muscle cells which causes the restenosis [66]. Further information on this is keenly awaited.

Conclusions

In summary, therefore, it would appear that the endothelium is extremely important in controlling, not only the diameter of coronary arteries, but also coronary vascular resistance. The factor derived from the endothelium may be the perfect autocoid, able to receive signals locally and be released locally, thus having its effect at that site. It may coordinate the aggregate hydrodynamic properties of an intact vascular network, and may oppose the positive feedback mechanism (the myogenic response) which, (if unopposed), could theoretically lead to instability in the intact circulation.

References

1. Buonassisi, V. Sulfated mucopolysaccharide synthesis and secretion in endothelial cell cultures. *Exp. Cell Res.*, **76**, 363–368, 1973
2. Chan, V. and Chan, T.K. Antithrombin III in fresh and cultured human endothelial cells. A natural anticoagulant from the vascular endothelium. *Thromb. Res.*, **15**, 209–213, 1979
3. Weksler, B.B., Eldor, A., Falcone, D., *et al.* Prostaglandins and vascular endothelium. In *Cardiovascular Pharmacology of the Prostaglandins* (eds A.G. Herman, P.M. Vanhoutte, and H. Denolin, *et al.*), Raven, New York, pp. 137–148, 1982
4. Loskutoff, D.J. and Edgington, T.S. Synthesis of a fibrinolytic activator and inhibitor by endothelial cells. *Proc. Natl. Acad. Sci. USA*, **74**, 3903–3907, 1977
5. Jaffe, E.A., Hoyer, L.W. and Nachman, R.L. Synthesis of von Willebrand factor by cultured human endothelial cells. *Proc. Natl. Acad. Sci. USA*, **71**, 1906–1909, 1974
6. Jaffe, E.A. and Mosher, D.F. Synthesis of fibronectin by cultured human endothelial cells. *Ann. NY Acad. Sci.*, **312**, 122–131, 1978
7. McPherson, J., Sage, H. and Bornstein, P. Isolation and characterisation of a glycoprotein secreted by aortic endothelial cells in culture. Apparent identity with platelet thrombospondin. *J. Biol. Chem.*, **256**, 11330–11336, 1981
8. Rorie, D.K. and Tyce, G.M. Uptake and metabolism of norepinephrine by endothelium of dog pulmonary artery. *Am. J. Physiol.*, **248**, H193–H197, 1985

9. Strux, J.M. and Jonod, A.F. Radioautographic demonstration of 5-hydroxytryptamine-³H uptake by pulmonary artery. *Am. J. Physiol.*, **248**, H193–H197, 1985

10. Pearson, J.D. and Gordon, J.L. Nucleotide metabolism by endothelium. *Ann. Rev. Physiol.*, **47**, 617–627, 1985

11. Ryan, U.S., Ryan, J.W., Whitaker, C., *et al.* Localisation of angiotensin converting enzyme (kininase II). II. Immunocytochemistry and immunofluorescence. *Tissue Cell*, **8**, 125–145, 1976

13. Furchgott, R.F. and Zawadzki, J.V. The obligatory role of endothelial cells in the relaxation of arterial smooth muscle by acetylcholine. *Nature (Lond.)*, **288**, 373–376, 1980

14. Furchgott, R.F. Role of endothelium in responses of vascular smooth muscle. *Circ. Res.*, **53**, 557–573, 1983

15. Cocks, T.M. and Angus, J.A. Endothelium-dependent relaxation of coronary arteries by noradrenaline and serotonin. *Nature (Lond.)*, **305**, 627–630, 1983

16. Saeed, M., Schmidli, J., Metz, M., *et al.* Perfused rabbit heart. Endothelium-derived relaxing factor in coronary arteries. *J. Cardiovasc. Pharmacol.*, **8**, 257–261, 1986

17. Holtz, J., Forstermann, U., Pohl, U., *et al.* Flow-dependent, endothelium-mediated dilation of epicardial coronary arteries in conscious dogs: effects of cyclooxygenase inhibition. *J. Cardiovasc. Pharmacol.*, **6**, 1161–1169, 1984

18. Rubanyi, G.M., Romero, J.C. and Vanhoutte, P.M. Flow-induced release of endothelium-derived relaxing factor. *Am. J. Physiol.*, **250**, H1145–H1149, 1986

19. Crossman, D., Larkin, S. and Davies, G. Substance P is a potent dilator of human epicardial vessels. *Eur. Heart J.*, **9 Suppl. 1**, 318:1775, 1988

20. McEwan, J., Larkin, S., Davies, G., *et al.* Calcitonin gene-related peptide: a potent dilator of human epicardial coronary arteries. *Circulation*, **74**, 1234–1237, 1986

21. Grace, G.C., Dusting, G.J., Kemp, B.E. and Martin, T.J. Endothelium and the vasodilator action of rat calcitonin gene-related peptide (CGRP). *Br. J. Pharmacol.*, **91**, 729–733, 1987

22. Ignarro, L.J., Byrns, R.E., Buga, G.M. and Wood, K.S. Mechanisms of endothelium-dependent vascular smooth muscle relaxation elicited by bradykinin and VIP. *Am. J. Physiol.*, **253**, H1074–1082, 1987

23. Kalsner, S. Cholinergic mechanisms in human coronary artery preparations: implications of species differences. *J. Physiol. Lond.*, **358**, 509–526, 1985

24. Ludmer, P.L., Selwyn, A.P., Shook, T.L., *et al.* Paradoxical vasoconstriction induced by acetylcholine in atherosclerotic coronary arteries. *N. Engl. J. Med.*, **315**, 1046–1051, 1986

25. Collins, P., Chappell, S.P., Griffith, T.M., *et al.* Differences in basal endothelium-derived relaxing factor activity in different artery types. *J. Cardiovasc. Pharmacol.*, **8**, 1158–1162, 1986

26. Martin, W., Villani, G.M., Jothianandan, D. and Furchgott, R.F. Selective blockade of endothelium-dependent and glycerul trinitrate-induced relaxation by haemoglobin and methylene blue in the rabbit aorta. *J. Pharmacol. Exp. Ther.*, **232**, 708–716, 1985

27. Bolin, R. and DeVenuto, F. Haemoglobin solutions as a blood substitute. In *Advances in Blood Substitute Research*, Alan R. Liss, New York, pp. 1–7, 1983

28. Fratantoni, J. Safety evaluation of haemoglobin solutions. In *Advances in Blood Substitute Research*, Alan R. Liss, New York, pp. 111–115, 1983

29. Palmer, R.M.J., Ferrige, A.G. and Moncada, S. Nitric oxide release accounts for the biological activity of endothelium-derived relaxing factor. *Nature (Lond.)*, **327**, 524–526, 1987

30. Myers, P.R., Minor, R.L., Jr., Guerra, R., *et al.* Vasorelaxant properties of the endothelium-derived relaxing factor more closely resemble S-nitrosocysteine than nitric oxide. *Nature (Lond.)*, **345**, 161–163, 1990

31. Pohl, U., Busse, R., Kuon, E. and Bassenge, E. Pulsatile perfusion stimulates the release of endothelial autocoids. *J. Appl. Cardiol.*, **1**, 1215–1235, 1986

32. Martin, W., Furchgott, R.F., Villani Gina, M. and Jothianandan, D. Phosphodiesterase inhibitors induce endothelium-dependent relaxation of rat and rabbit aorta by potentiating the effects of spontaneously released endothelium-derived relaxing factor. *J. Pharmacol. Exp. Ther.*, **237**, 539–547, 1986

33. Edwards, D.H., Griffith, T.M., Ryley, H.C. and Henderson, A.H. Haptoglobin–haemoglobin complex in human plasma inhibits endothelium-dependent relaxation: evidence that endothelium-derived relaxing factor acts as a local autocoid. *Cardiovasc. Res.*, **20**, 549–556, 1986

34. Azuma, H., Ishikawa, M. and Sekizaki, S. Endothelium-dependent inhibition of platelet aggregation. *Br J. Pharmacol.*, **88**, 411–415, 1986

35. Furlong, B., Henderson, A.H., Lewis, M.J. and Smith, J.A. Endothelium-derived relaxing factor inhibits *in vitro* platelet aggregation. *Br. J. Pharmacol.*, **90**, 687–692, 1987

36. Radomski. M.W., Palmer, R.M.J. and Moncada, S. Endogenous nitric oxide inhibits human platelet adhesion to vascular endothelium. *Lancet*, **ii**, 1057–1058, 1987

37. Hogan, J.C., Lewis, M.J. and Henderson, A.H. *In vivo* EDRF activity influences platelet function. *Br. J. Pharmacol.*, **94**, 1020–1022, 1988
38. Chappell, S.P., Lewis, M.J. and Henderson, A.H. Effect of lipid feeding on endothelium dependent relaxation in rabbit aortic preparations. *Cardiovasc. Res.*, **21**, 34–38, 1987
39. Freiman, P.C., Mitchell, G.G., Heistad, D.D., *et al.* Atherosclerosis impairs endothelium-dependent vascular relaxation to acetylcholine and thrombin in primates. *Circ. Res.*, **58**, 783–789, 1986
40. Ginsburg, R. and Zera, P.H. Endothelial relaxant factor in the human epicardial coronary artery. *Circulation*, **70 (Suppl. II)**, 122, 1984
41. Coene, M.C. and Herman, A.G. Effect of hypercholesterolemia on vascular reactivity in the rabbit: 1: Endothelium-dependent and endothelium-independent contractions and relaxation in isolated arteries of control and hypercholesterolemic rabbits. *Circ. Res.*, **58**, 552–564, 1986
42. Senaratne, M. Endothelium-dependent relaxation (EDR) and experimental atherosclerosis. *J. Mol. Cell. Cardiol.*, **18 (Suppl. 3)**, 38 (abstract), 1986
43. Habib, J.B., Bossaller, C., Wells, S., *et al.* Preservation of endothelium-dependent relaxation vascular relaxation in cholesterol-fed rabbits by treatment with the calcium blocker PN 200110. *Circ. Res.*, **58**, 305–309, 1986
44. Harrison, D.G., Armstrong, M.L., Freiman, P.C. and Heistad, D.D. Restoration of endothelium-dependent relaxation by dietary treatment of atherosclerosis, *J. Clin. Invest.*, **80**, 1808–1811, 1987
45. Shimokawa, H., Lam, J.Y.T., Chesebro, J.G., *et al.* Effects of dietary supplementation with cod-liver oil on endothelium-dependent response in porcine coronary arteries. *Circulation*, **76**, 898–905, 1987
46. Van de Voorde, J. and Jeusen, I. Endothelium-dependent and independent relaxation of aortic rings from hypertensive rats. *Am. J. Physiol.*, **250**, H711–717, 1986
47. Cabbiani, C.T., Elemer, G., Guelpa, C., *et al.* Morphologic and functional changes of the aortic intima during experimental hypertension. *Am. J. Pathol.*, **96**, 399–422, 1979
48. Dole, W.P., Lamping, K.G. and Marcus, M.L. Endothelium and large coronary artery response to 5-hydroxytryptamine *in vivo*. *Blood Vessels*, **23**, 64 (abstract), 1986
49. Miller, M.L., Pinto, A. and Mullane, K.M. Impaired endothelium-dependent relaxations in rabbits subjected to aortic coarction hypertension. *Hypertension*, **10**, 164–170, 1987
50. Vallance, P., Collier, J. and Moncada, S. Effects of endothelium-derived nitric oxide on peripheral anteriolar tone in man. *Lancet*, **ii**, 997–1000, 1989
51. Maseri, A., Chierchia, S., Davies, G.J., *et al.* Variable susceptibility to dynamic coronary obstruction: An elusive link between coronary atherosclerosis and angina pectoris. *Am. J. Cardiol.*, **52**, 46A–51A, 1983
52. Pomerance, A. Peri-arterial mast cells in coronary atheroma and thrombosis. *J. Pathol. Bacteriol.*, **76**, 55–70, 1958
53. Forman, M.B., Oates, J.A., Robertson, D., *et al.* Increased adventitial mast cells in a patient with coronary spasm. *N. Engl. J. Med.*, **313**, 1138–1141, 1985
54. Weiss, L. and Löffler, G. Interrelationship between adipose tissue and liver. *Hormone Metab. Res.*, **S2**, 196–203, 1970
55. Hennig, B., Shasby, D.M. and Spector, A.A. Exposure to fatty acid increases human low density lipoprotein transfer across cultured endothelial monolayers. *Circ. Res.*, **57**, 776–780, 1985
56. Vanhoutte, P.M. and Houston, D.S. Platelets, endothelium, and vasospasm. *Circulation*, **5**, 728–734, 1985
57. Bossaller, C., Yamamoto, H., Lichtlen, P.R. and Henry, P.D. Impaired cholinergic vasodilation in the cholesterol-fed rabbit *in vivo*. *Basic Res. Cardiol.*, **82**, 396–404, 1987
58. Crea, F., Davies, G., Chierchia, S., *et al.* Different susceptibility to myocardial ischemia provoked by hyperventilation and cold pressure test in exertional and variant angina pectoris. *Am. J. Cardiol.*, **56**, 18–22, 1985
59. Maseri, A., Chierchia, S. and Kaski, J.C. Mixed angina pectoris. *Am. J. Cardiol.*, **56**, 30E–33E, 1985
60. Falk, E. Plaque rupture with severe pre-existing stenosis precipitating coronary thrombosis: Characteristics of coronary atherosclerotic plaques underlying fatal occlusive thrombi. *Br. Heart J.*, **50**, 127–132, 1983
61. Davies, M.J. and Thomas, A. Thrombosis and acute coronary-artery lesions in sudden cardiac ischemic death. *N. Engl. J. Med.*, **310**, 1137–1142, 1984
62. Maseri, A., Chierchia, S. and Davies, G. Pathophysiology of coronary occlusion in acute infarction. *Circulation*, **73**, 233–239, 1986
63. Kalsner, S. and Richards, R. Coronary arteries of cardiac patients are hyperreactive and contain stores of amines: A mechanism for coronary spasm. *Science*, **223**, 1435–1437, 1984
64. Cowley, M.J., Vetrovec, G.W. and Wolfgang, T.C. Efficacy of percutaneous transluminal coronary

angioplasty: Technique, patient selection, salutary results, limitations and complications. *Am. Heart J.*, **101**, 272–280, 1981

65. Kent, K.M., Bentivoglio, L.G., Block, P.C., *et al.* Percutaneous transluminal coronary angioplasty: Report from the registry of the national heart, lung and blood institute. *Am. J. Cardiol.*, **49**, 2011–2020, 1982

66. Garg, U.C., Hassid, A. Nitric oxide-generating vasodilators and 8-bromo-cyclic guanosine monophosphate inhibit mitogenesis and proliferation of cultured rat vascular smooth muscle cells. . *Clin. Invest.*, **83**, 1774–1777, 1989

11

Molecular and cellular changes in ventricular hypertrophy and failure

P. Pauletto, G. Vescovo, L. Dalla Libera, G. Scannapieco,
A.C. Pessina, C. Dal Palŭ, P.A. Poole-Wilson and S.E. Harding

Introduction

The ventricle responds to chronic overload by increasing the mass of contractile elements to normalize wall stress[1]. It is assumed that chronic pressure overload results in parallel addition of new myofibrils (patterns of concentric hypertrophy) while chronic volume overload leads to addition of new sarcomeres in series (patterns of eccentric hypertrophy)[2]. Although this remodelling of the ventricular chamber allows apparent normal myocardial function over long periods, the chronic overload inevitably leads to hemodynamic failure. Ventricular hypertrophy cannot be regarded just as a quantitative process accompanied by changes in ventricular geometry. Remodelling of the myocardium in response to sustained stress takes place at extracellular, cellular and molecular levels. These changes enable the heart to meet the altered demand, until decompensation occurs through mechanisms which have not been fully elucidated. This review summarizes some of our findings concerning the molecular and cellular changes occurring in both compensated and decompensated ventricular hypertrophy. Changes in the isozymes of creatine kinase and myosin are described. The contractile characteristics of single muscle cells isolated from hypertrophied or failing ventricles are related to changes in composition of the isozymes. Single myocytes are also used to investigate the basic muscle contractility of the failing heart, and the adaptation of the cascade from beta-adrenoceptors to adenylate cyclase. At all stages, we emphasize the relevance of animal models to the investigation of human disease.

Glycolysis and mitochondrial activity

An increased glycolytic activity has been reported in cardiac hypertrophy and in congestive failure[3]. Lactate dehydrogenase, a specific enzyme in anaerobic metabolism, is also increased[4]. The M tetramer of lactate dehydrogenase, which is nearly absent in the normal heart, increases during chronic pressure overload in different animal models as well as in humans. The pathophysiological significance of this finding remains to be fully elucidated. It may well be related to growth of non-muscle cells, such as fibroblasts, that are rich in M tetramer. In general, the increase in the anaerobic glycolysis can be viewed as an adaptive process to the reduced supply of oxygen, this reflecting the inadequate vascular growth of the hypertrophic myocardium.

Conflicting reports exist in the literature about changes in mitochondria from hypertrophic and failing hearts. This is likely to be due to the different types of animal models studied, the duration and severity of hypertrophy and/or failure, the mitochondrial preparations, and the biochemical assays used. The main question (whether or not changes in mitochondrial activity represent a primary causative factor in heart failure) has not yet been satisfactorily answered. It is clear, none the less, that changes in mitochondrial volume and function occur during the progression from the early stages of hypertrophy toward failure.

Morphological studies have shown that, as ventricular hypertrophy progresses, both the ratio of mitochondrial to cell volume and that of mitochondria to myofibrillar volume decrease[5–7]. Studies both in experimental models and in humans have shown that, during the early stage of pressure induced hypertrophy, the ratio of oxygen to adenosine diphosphate, and the quotient of oxygen in State 3 (QO_2^3) (which are the basic parameters of the mitochondrial respiratory activity) are markedly increased[8]. When the degree of hypertrophy is stable, respiratory activity begins to decline. When failure occurs, mitochondria exhibit a fall in both parameters of activity, indicating that a depression in respiratory activity has occurred along with an impairment in efficiency of synthesis of adenosine triphosphate[8,9]. The synthesis of mitochondrial cytochromes throughout the above mentioned stages of pressure-overload hypertrophy also shows a similar pattern[10]. All these changes at the mitochondrial level represent only a small part of the processes that regulate the energy supply to myofibrils. Together with changes in the creatine-kinase system, they may account for the decrease in both creatine phosphate and adenosine triphosphate described in the hypertrophic ventricles.

The creatine-kinase system

Ingwall and co-workers have shown a change in the distribution of isoenzymic forms of creatine kinase in the hypertrophied ventricles of spontaneously hypertensive rats, dogs, and patients with aortic stenosis. In man, this redistribution is accompanied by significant decrease in total activity of creatine kinase[11,12]. A marked reduction in levels of both creatine phosphate and adenosine triphosphate has also been reported in patients with ventricular hypertrophy. Creatine kinase is a dimeric enzyme (84 000 daltons) that catalyses the transfer of high-energy phosphate between adenosine diphosphate and creatine. In the rat ventricular myocardium, at least four electro-phoretically distinct isoenzymes exist: BB, MB, MM, and mitochondrial. There are conflicting data on the composition of isoenzymes in the normal human myocardium. Some authors report[13,14] the existence of the BB isoenzyme, while others do not find this isoform in human myocardium[12,15,16].

The mitochondrial creatine kinase produces creatine phosphate that is utilized by myofibrils for contraction and is used on membranes for transport of ions. In spontaneously hypertensive rats, renovascular hypertensive rats and in rats with aortic stenosis, a significant shift occurs toward the BB and MB forms[11,17,18]. This shift is directly related to the degree of cardiac hypertrophy[18]. An increase in the B monomer of creatine kinase at the expense of the M variety is aso found in patients with compensated aortic stenosis, both in the presence and in the absence of ischaemic heart disease[12]. Since the rate of reaction of the BB isoform in the presence of creatine phosphate and adenosine triphosphate is much slower than that of the MM form[19], it is conceivable that the shift toward the B monomer occurring in cardiac hypertrophy may lead to increased storage of energy as creatine phosphate. Moreover, the Michaelis constant of the BB isoform for both adenosine triphosphate and creatine is much lower than that of the MB and MM variants[20]. This means that, in the hypertrophied myocardium, the affinity for substrates is much higher, resulting in better utilization of the substrates themselves. These changes are thought to have an adaptational meaning and, possibly, to delay the occurrence of failure. Few data on human myocardium, however, are available in the literature[12,21]. We studied the activity and the isoenzyme distribution of creatine kinase in hearts from patients undergoing cardiac transplantation for dilated cardiomyopathies.

Ten to 20 mg samples of myocardium were homogenized at 4°C in 0.1 mmol/l potassium phosphate buffer, pH 7.4, containing EDTA 1 mmol/l and 1 beta-mercaptoethanol 1 mmol/l. The protein concentration was determined by the method of Lowry et al.[22] Total creatine kinase activity was measured according to the guidelines of the German Society for Clinical Chemistry[23] by using the Merck CK-NAC (Merck Darmstadt Germany). The distribution of the four creatine-kinase isoenzymes was determined by measurement of the creatine phosphate-dependent colorimetric reaction after electrophoretic separation of isoenzymes. The electrophoresis was carried out at 180 V for 25 minutes by using cellulose-acetate strips embedded in barbital buffer (pH 8.3–8.7). The concentration of substrates was not limiting for any of the isoenzymes in that they were assayed under the same conditions used for the measurement of total creatine kinase activity. The relative amount of each isoenzyme was determined by densitometric measurement of the electrophoretic bands at 550 nm. Total creatine-kinase activity expressed as IU/mg tissue was lower in ventricles and septums from patients with dilated cardiomyopathy than in control samples (Table 11.1). It was even lower when expressed as IU/mg of non-collagen protein (Table 11.2), suggesting a more marked decrease at the level of the contractile elements than in the whole tissue. The values found for the control samples are among the highest reported in the literature for the normal ventricular myocardium. Total activity of creatine kinase of normal ventricular myocardium varies from 0.5 to 14.7 IU/mg protein[24], depending on several methodological factors.

Samples from the atrial walls from patients with dilated cardiomyopathies gave lower values of total activity than those taken from the ventricles. A similar finding has been described by Bendz et al.[15] in hearts from patients who underwent replacement of the mitral valve. Since few data are available on normal human atria, it is difficult to understand the significance of such a difference between atria and

Table 11.1 Total creatine kinase activity (IU/mg tissue) in the heart of patients suffering from idiopathic dilated cardiomyopathy and of normal subjects

Normal subjects		Idiopathic dilated cardiomyopathy				
LV	Septum	Septum	LV	RV	LA	RA
1.72	1.61	—	1.13	1.03	0.97	0.22
—	1.31	1.19	1.68	1.58	0.83	0.81
		—	1.45	1.19	0.57	1.11
Mean			1.42	1.27	0.79	0.71
SD			0.28	0.28	0.20	0.45

LV = Left ventricle; RV = right ventricle; LA = left atrium; RA = right atrium.

Table 11.2 Total creatine kinase activity (IU/mg protein) in the heart of patients suffering from idiopathic dilated cardiomyopathy and of normal subjects

Normal subjects		Idiopathic dilated cardiomyopathy				
LV	Septum	Septum	LV	RV	LA	RA
16.6	14.5	–	12.8	10.3	9.2	8.1
–	10.9	7.2	9.8	10.7	10.2	6.5
		–	5.6	5.0	4.7	6.6
Mean			9.4	8.6	8.0	7.0
SD			3.6	3.1	2.9	0.9

LV = Left ventricle; RV = right ventricle; LA = left atrium; RA = right atrium.

ventricles. The decrease in total activity of creatine kinase that we have found in the ventricles of patients with dilated cardiomyopathies appears similar to that previously described for cardiac hypertrophy and failure[11,12]. A larger number of normal control samples would give further significance to our observations. We do not know whether the decrease in total activity of creatine kinase plays a pathogenetic role in ventricular failure. It may, instead, be a common adaptive feature of both compensated cardiac hypertrophy and idiopathic dilated cardiomyopathies.

Distribution of isoenzymes of creatine kinase in patients with dilated cardiomyopathies is characterized by a decrease in both MM and mitochondrial forms. This reduction is counterbalanced by an increase in the MB isoform (Figure 11.1). There is, however, a high variability within normal subjects. This is, in part, due to the difficulty of separating electrophoretically the mitochondrial band in humans. Some authors also describe the existence of other forms in the human enzymic system[14] and suggest the inadequacy of the M-B dimeric model to describe the system of creatine-kinase isoforms[13]. In particular, the presence of variants of the mitochon-

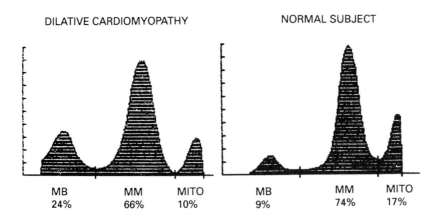

DILATIVE CARDIOMYOPATHY   NORMAL SUBJECT

MB	MM	MITO	MB	MM	MITO
24%	66%	10%	9%	74%	17%

TOTAL CK ACTIVITY: 16.6 IU/mg prot   TOTAL CK ACTIVITY: 9.8 IU/mg prot

Figure 11.1 Representative electrophoretograms of creatine kinase isoforms from homogenates of left ventricle. The cathode is to the right. MITO = mitochondrial form

drial fraction has been reported for the normal human myocardium[14], together with the expression of small amounts of the BB isoform[13,14]. Other studies, carried out with similar methods to those that we have used, showed no variants in mitochondrial fraction and no presence of the BB isoform[12,15,16]. Such discrepancies will probably be clarified by using monoclonal antibodies or immunoblotting techniques. The increase of the MB isoform, with parallel decrease of the MM one found in our parients, is similar to that described for the hypertrophied, non-failing human myocardium[12]. It is likely to have an adaptive significance. On the other hand, a decrease in mitochondrial form as observed in our patients has been reported for hypertrophied or failing rat hearts[11,15]. This could reflect the decrease in the fractional volume of mitochondria described in failure. The present data, together with previous animal studies, suggest that a decrease in mitochondrial form associated with a decrease in total activity of creatine kinase is the hallmark of the transition from compensated hypertrophy to failure.

Synthesis of collagen

Protein synthesis, measured by the incorporation of labelled lysine, increases a few hours after the imposition of pressure overload, while protein degradation slows down[26]. At the same time, an increased rate of synthesis occurs both in RNA and in DNA-dependent RNA polymerase[27]. In some experimental models, the increased rate of synthesis can lead to a significant increase in heart weight within 24–48 hours. It has been reported that the rate of incorporation of amino acids into protein, normalized for the amount of RNA, is increased[28]. This means that the efficiency of protein synthesis is enhanced. Though myofibrillar protein synthesis is predominant in the early phases of cardiac hypertrophy, in the subsequent stages the collagen fraction also increases, The myocytes are embedded in a matrix of connective tissue which helps to maintain both cell-to-cell and cell-to-capillary geometry. The collagenous network is composed by myocyte-to-myocyte and the myocyte-to-capillary struts which are similar in diameter (about 150 nm) and number[29]. Weaves of collagen strands surround groups of myocytes, and adjacent weaves are connected by tendon-like processes[29]. The extracellular matrix of the myocardium consists of other components than collagen, but these are much more difficult to evaluate. The collagenous struts are thought to ensure the maintenance of ventricular geometry during diastole as well as capillary patency during systole. The extracellular matrix is a dynamic tissue and responds rapidly to the increased working load[30]. The collagenous matrix is usually evaluated by morphometric methods (surface measurements; electron microscopy) and/or by assay of hydroxyproline levels. Morphometric approaches have shown that both types of strut can double in diameter in human hypertensive heart disease[31].

Sometimes a distortion may occur in the weave. Such a change may, at least in part, explain the variability in ventricular stiffness observed in hearts subjected to similar strain[31]. Morphometric studies have shown that collagen increases by about 30% in hypertrophied, non-failing hearts from hypertensive patients, and by about 80% in hearts from hypertensive patients with overt failure[32]. In hypertensive rats, the content of hydroxyproline in the subendocardial layer is higher than in the subepicardial one, suggesting that synthesis of collagen starts in the subendocardium[33]. This observation, however, has not been confirmed in humans, at least with morphological techniques[34]. Inappropriate growth of myocardial collagen may lead to encirling of individual myocytes and capillaries with reduction of their anatomical and functional area. It may also alter conduction, producing delayed or late potentials. The increase in collagenous matrix observed in the hypertrophic myocardium may also, by increasing ventricular stiffness, contribute to the change in the viscoelastic properties of the heart. It is worth noting that only preliminary data are available on the physiological role of the different phenotypes of cardiac collagen. The significance of these changes in pathological conditions is still obscure[35].

Characteristics of muscle cells

The study of single muscle cells isolated from the ventricles of failing or hypertrophied hearts can help to distinguish between changes in basic contractility and alterations due to increased synthesis of collagen. We have developed techniques for the isolation of viable, contracting myocytes from the atria or ventricles of human and animal hearts[36–38]. The individual cells thus obtained are placed in a bath on the stage of an inverted microscope, warmed to 32°C and electrically stimulated at 0.2 Hz (human ventricle) or 0.5 Hz (human atria, animal atria or ventricle). The image of a single beating cell is captured using a video camera and the change in length with each beat (contraction amplitude) is displayed continuously on a paper chart recorder. The velocity of contraction and relaxation are also continuously recorded.

A large amount of preliminary work has been aimed at investigating the validity of the use of single cells to make deductions about the condition of the heart from which they were isolated. Heterogeneity of isolated myocytes, either intrinsic or caused by the isolation procedure, might, in theory, limit the value of the method applied to tissue of failing hearts. This has not been so in animal experiments. We have shown that species-dependent properties of velocity of contraction and relaxation are retained in single ventricular cells, as are differences from those obtained from the right and left ventricles[38]. Decreases in isotonic shortening demonstrated in the cardiomyopathic ventricle have been observed in myocytes isolated from the ventricular tissue[39]. Changes in velocity during hypertrophy and failure are detected at the level of the single cell, and correlate with shifts in the isoforms of ventricular myosin[40]. Contractile responses to beta-adrenoceptor agonists and other inotropic agents are preserved, and the variability between cells and between animals is similar to that described for muscle strips[36]. Exposure of the whole animal to high levels of catecholamine produces a desensitization of beta-adrenoceptor response that is detectable in the individual myocyte[41]. It is as homogeneous in cells as it is in papillary muscles[42]. Analysis of variance shows that a number of cells from one patient or one animal have similar characteristics. This is an important prerequisite for any claim that single cells can be representative of whole muscle.

The basic contractile characteristics of myocytes from failing and non-failing human hearts have been studied by investigating the contraction amplitude, and velocity of contraction of relaxation, in a maximally activating concentration of extracellular calcium.

Human ventricular tissue was obtained from explanted hearts at the time of transplant or during routine cardiac surgery. Eleven of the patients (22 male and 7 female, mean (ISD) age 43.8 ± 18.4 years, range 7–76) had ischaemic heart disease, 8 congenital abnormalities, 4 mitral valvar disease, 4 congestive cardiomyopathy and two viral myocarditis. Two hearts that were originally from normal donors were obtained during heart–lung retransplant performed due to rejection of the lungs.

Pieces of ventricle (100 mg to 3 g) were chopped quickly into chunks of approximately 1 mm³ using an array of razor blades. The chunks were incubated for a total of 12 min at 35°C in 25–50 ml of a low calcium medium (LC) of the following composition: (in mmol/l) NaCl 120, KCl 5.4, MgSO$_4$ 5, pyruvate 5, glucose 20, taurine 20, HEPES 10, nitrilotriacetic acid 5, pH 6.96, containing 1–2 μmmol/l calcium. The medium was changed three times during this period. The chunks were stirred by bubbling with 100% O$_2$. The low calcium medium was removed by straining with 300μm gauze. The chunks were then incubated at 35°C for 45 min in the above solution with nitrilotriacetic acid omitted and 4 U/ml (Sigma) type XXIV protease (pronase) and 30 μmol/l calcium added, followed by two 45 min periods with the protease omitted and 400 IU/ml (BCL) collagenase added. The medium was shaken gently throughout the incubation, and kept under an atmosphere of 100% O$_2$. At the end of the second and third 45 min periods the solution containing the dispersed cells was filtered through a 300 μm gauze and centrifuged at 40 g min^{-1} for 1–2 min. The cells were washed twice by centrifugation in Krebs–Henseleit medium (in mmol/l): NaCl 119, KCl 4.7, MgSO$_4$ 0.94, KH$_2$PO$_4$ 1.2, NaHCO$_3$ 25, glucose 11.5, containing 1 or 1.3 mmol/l calcium and equilibrated to pH 7.4 with 95% O$_2$, 5% CO$_2$, and resuspended in the same medium.

There is no single simple measure of the severity of heart failure. We have, therefore, used several indicators of the severity of disease which could readily be obtained in most patients. These were the New York Heart Association classification of symptoms of breathlessness, the left ventricular ejection fraction, the left ventricular end diastolic pressure and the amount of diuretics prescribed. This latter was divided into classes:

1. No diuretic.
2. Frusemide 20 mg daily or a thiazide diuretic.
3. Frusemide 40 mg.
4. Frusemide 80 mg.
5. Greater than 120 mg frusemide.

The maximum contraction amplitude (percentage cell shortening) in response to increasing extracellular calcium was not correlated with any indicator of disease. This was true for both pooled and non-pooled data, and for cells from both right and left ventricles (Figure 11.2). Some trends to a difference between aetiologies were evident in absolute contraction amplitude in high calcium, with cells from patients with congenital heart disease giving a larger percentage shortening (12.1 ± 0.74%m n = 12) than those with congestive cardiomyopathy (8.9 ± 0.5%, n = 11, p < 0.01, non-pooled data). The patients with congenital abnormalities, however, tended to be younger. The relation between age and aetiology is discussed more fully below.

Velocities for individual cells were measured in two ways. First, the maximum rate of contraction or relaxation was continuously displayed on the chart trace at the same time as the amplitude. These parameters will increase as the amplitude increases if the time-to-peak-shortening or relaxation remains unaltered. Second, the time to peak shortening, time to 50% relaxation, and time to 90% relaxation were measured from the trace at the point of maximum contraction amplitude, before signs of toxicity were evident, for either calcium or isoprenaline.

There was no relation between the severity of disease, as defined by New York Heart Association class, left ventricular ejection fraction, left ventricular end diastolic

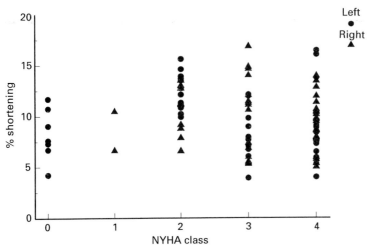

Figure 11.2 Contraction amplitude of individual myocytes in high calcium. Relation to NYHA class of symptoms of the patient

pressure or diuretic class and the parameters of contraction measured in maximum calcium. Nor was there any clear association between aetiology of disease and velocities of contraction or relaxation in high calcium. This was true for pooled or non-pooled data, and for cells from both the right and left ventricles.

When the data were analysed according to the age of the patient, however, significant changes in basic contractility were seen. A different pattern of change with age was evident in right and left ventricular cells. Maximum amplitude (percentage shortening) did not change with age in left ventricular myocytes, but the times to both 50% and 90% of relaxation were significantly slowed in cells from older patients (Figure 11.3). In cells from the right ventricle, the maximum amplitude decreased significantly with increasing age ($n = 58$, $r = 0.30$, $p < 0.02$), as did the maximum rates of contraction ($n = 48$, $r = 0.33$, $p < 0.05$) and relaxation ($n = 49$, $r = 0.37$, $p < 0.01$). The other parameters of contraction were unaffected in right ventricular cells.

These results suggest that there is little relation between the severity of disease and the impairment in basic contractile function of the individual cells. The results for maximum amplitude are in agreement with those of other groups, who have found that papillary muscles from the failing human heart are able to generate the same amount of tension as non-failing ones[43–45]. There are reports, however, of prolonged contraction and relaxation, as well as extended transients of calcium in muscle from failing human hearts[44,46], notably when hypertrophy is present. Although the overall changes in relaxation in our studies were not significant, cells from some patients showed abnormally extended times to 50% and 90% relaxation. These patients were suffering from dilated or hypertrophic cardiomyopathy. More data from patients in these groups is required before any conclusions can be drawn. The lack of change of relaxation time in the isolated myocytes from the ventricles of patients with ischaemic heart disease could be due to a number of factors. The slowing of whole muscle contraction may be related to changes in fibrous tissue, as discussed above. Alternatively, the limitations of the use of isolated cells could

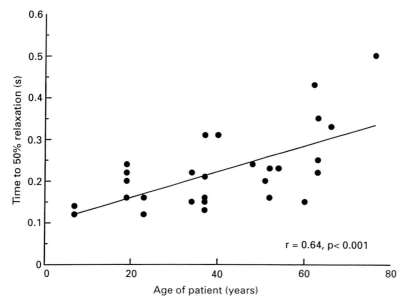

Figure 11.3 Variation of contractile parameters with age of the patient. Time to 50% relaxation in maximum calcium, left ventricular cells, n = 29 cells (16 patients)

prevent observation of these changes, either because the most vigorously contracting cells are preferentially selected for study, or because they are studied under conditions of minimum load. A third possibility is that the alterations in the intact muscle related more to the age of the patient than cardiac failure, since they are similar to those we have observed for cells from ageing muscle. Fourth, the changes seen in whole muscle[44,46] may be a consequence of hypertrophy rather than failure.

Contractile proteins

The changes in energy metabolism and mechanics so far reported in hypertrophied hearts are related largely to structural changes in specific contractile proteins. Indeed, evidence has grown about the regulatory role played by the expression of different isoforms of cardiac myosin. Changes in other contractile proteins, like actin, tropomyosin and troponin, seem not to play a major role. Preliminary studies described the existence of different isoforms of actin[47] and of troponin, the role of which in hypertrophy has not yet been clarified. Also, a new tropomyosin appears in hypertrophied rat ventricles. This differs in primary structure from tropmyosin observed in normal animals[48]. The pathophysiological significance of such a change remains obscure. Conversely, myosin represents the main myocardial contractile protein because, in most mammalian species, both contractile properties[49] and oxygen consumption[50] of the myocardium depend on the composition of the myosin heavy chain. Myosin has a hexameric structure consisting of two heavy chains and two pairs of light chains (light chain 1 and light chain 2) in the 200 000 and 20 000 dalton molecular weight range, respectively.

Various isoforms of both light and heavy chains are known to occur. Two types of myosin heavy chains, alpha and beta respectively, exist in cardiac muscle. These two types of heavy chains are combined, forming an alpha–alpha homodimer, an alpha–beta heterodimer, or a beta–beta homodimer, which correspond to the V_1, V_2 and V_3 isoforms originally described by Hoh et al.[51]. Young normotensive male rats always show a polymorphic pattern of ventricular myosin, with prevalence of the V_1 isoform (about 70%) over V_2 and V_3 (15% each)[52]. In studies carried out by our group, and others using immunohistochemical[53] and electrophoretic[54] methods, it has been shown that the development of both pressure- and volume-induced cardiac hypertrophy is paralleled by a shift from V_1 toward V_2 and V_3 isomyosins. The V_3 isoform is characterized by low speed of muscle shortening calcium-activated ATPase, and consumption of oxygen, resulting in an improved economy of generation of force[55]. V_1 has opposite characteristics and V_2 has intermediate properties. As a consequence, the shift toward the V_3 isoform occurring both in spontaneously[56] and renovascular hypertensive rats[57] with progression of cardiac hypertrophy is regarded as beneficial and of adaptational significance. It allows the myocardium to maintain its pumping function and, at the same time, to save energy[57]. When the stable phase of cardiac hypertrophy is reached in rats rendered hypertensive by clipping one renal artery, the percentage of V_3 isomyosin in the left ventricle is closely correlated to the degree of cardiac hypertrophy[58]. Several other pathophysiologic stimuli (and also some antihypertensive drugs) are able to modify the patterns of ventricular isomyosins in both normotensive and hypertensive rats. Ageing[52], hypothyroidism[51], diabetes[59], gonadectomy[60], and high sodium intake[61] lead to a shift toward the isoenzyme V_3 with low ATPase activity. In contrast, hyperthyroidism[51], increased catecholamines levels[62], and swimming training[63] bring about a preferential synthesis of the isoenzyme V_1 with high ATPase activity.

As a general rule[52,57], small mammals such as rats, rabbits, and guinea pigs show a polymorphic pattern of ventricular myosin, with prevalence of the V_1 isomyosin. The decreased velocity of muscle shortening occurring in cardiac overload as a consequence of the shift toward V_3 has a beneficial effect. Moreover, in spontaneously hypertensive turkeys, which display high levels of catecholamines, we found that cardiac hypertrophy develops with synthesis of 'fast' V_1-like myosin and is accompanied by early decompensation[64]. We have studied the composition of myosin isoforms and the contraction amplitude and velocity of single ventricular myocytes from an animal model of hypertrophy, the monocrotaline-treated rat. Monocrotaline, a pyrrolizidine alkaloid, causes a severe pulmonary hypertension when given intraperitoneally. This results in a selective right ventricular hypertrophy. Ratios of weight of the right ventricle and body were increased by a factor of three, whereas the ratios of the left ventricle and body weight ratios were unchanged.

Male Sprague–Dawley rats of weight 75–100 g were injected intraperitoneally with monocrotaline (30 mg/kg). Treated rats were allowed to eat freely from a supply of standard rat cubes. Control rats were injected with saline and diet-matched to the treated rats by allowing them only the quantity of food consumed on the previous day by the treated rats. After an initial phase of mortality due to liver damage, a second phase occurred, thought to be due to cardiac failure secondary to pulmonary hypertension. About half of the surviving rats showed severe right ventricular hypertrophy and pleural, pericardial and peritoneal effusions. The remainder continued to eat well but were subsequently found to have severe right ventricular hypertrophy. At 3 weeks after monocrotaline treatment, when the first phase of mortality was over, some groups of rats were put in metabolic cages to allow measurement every 24 h of food and water intake and urine volume. Animals were used for isolation of cardiac mycocytes in an order dictated by the severity of their symptoms, beginning with those judges to be about to enter the second phase of mortality described above, followed by the remainder which continued to eat well. Criteria used to suggest severe illness of the rats were decreased food and water intakes and urine output as well as laboured breathing and more general characteristics such as poor condition of fur.

Purification of myosin was carried out from a 10–15 mg pellet of isolated cells obtained by centrifugation at 10 000 g for 10 min of a sample of the first digest. We processed 10 samples from the right ventricle and 11 samples from the left ventricle of the monocrotaline-treated animals. In the control animals seven samples from the right ventricle and seven from the left were studied. Samples were processed for myosin purification according to previously described procedures[65]. The protein concentration was determined by the method of Lowry[22]. Myosin Ca^{2+}-activated ATPase activity was assayed as previously described[65]. The assay mixture contained KCl 25 mmol-l, $CaCl_2$ 10 mmol/l, adenosine triphosphate 2.5 mmol/l and Tris HCl 50 mmol/l, pH 7.6. The protein concentration was 0.1 mg/ml in a final volume of 1 ml. The reaction was carried out at 25°C for 5 minutes beginning with the addition of adenosine triphosphate. The liberated inorganic phosphate was measured as described by Lanzetta et al.[66]. Two-dimensional polyacrylamide gel-electrophoresis of myosin light chains was carried out according to O'Farrell[67].

Both the Ca^{2+}-ATPase activity, and the proportion of alpha-chain myosin were decreased in the hypertrophied right ventricle but not in the left. The electrophoretic analysis confirmed the shift in myosin isoforms from mainly VI towards a mixture of V1, V2 and V3. Cells from the hypertrophied ventricle showed a significantly decreased velocity of contraction compared with controls. There was a significant correlation between the myosin alpha-chain percentage for the ventricle and the speed of shortening of an individual myocyte isolated from that ventricle. This was true when cells were activated maximally by either isoprenaline ($r = 0.72$, $p < 0.01$, Figure 11.4) or calcium ($r = 0.52$, $p < 0.05$)[40]. These results show that the measurement of parameters of contraction of individual cells can reflect changes that have taken place within the whole ventricle. The reason that we were unable to detect similar changes in myocytes from hypertrophied human heart is unlikely to be due to the technique, and is probably more related to the differences in adaptation between large and small animals.

Large mammals (such as cows, pigs and man) possess a pattern of ventricular myosin mainly composed of beta heavy chains, with the consequent prevalence of V_3 [57,68]. For this reason, humans do not have the same adaptational capacity as small mammals. A decrease in contractility in the hypertrophied myocardium implies impending decompensation[57]. It has been suggested that a possible adaptive mechanism takes place in humans at the level of the myosin light chains, which influence activity of myofibrillar adenosine triphosphatase. Hirzel et al.[69] found that in both volume- and pressure-overloaded human ventricles as well as in ventricles from patients with idiopathic dilated cardiomyopathy, an additional atrial-like light chain 1 appears. This author reported that the amounts of this additional light chain myosin correlated with the values of mean peak circumferential wall stress. Moreover, the expression of this additional myosin light chain was enhanced in

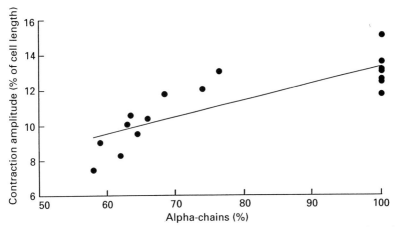

Figure 11.4 Correlation between alpha-chain percentage of the whole ventricle and speed of shortening of individual cells from control (alpha-chains % = 100) and monocrotaline-treated rats (right ventricle) (from reference[40], by permission.)

patients with dilated cardiomyopathy and during the earlier stages of ventricular hypertrophy[69]. We have studied samples of myocardium taken from patients who underwent cardiac transplantation for chronic heart failure due to dilated cardiomyopathy.

Myosin light chain pattern and Ca^{2+}-activated ATPase activity were studied in full-thickness samples taken from ventricles and atria of 8 patients undergoing cardiac transplantation for idiopathic dilated cardiomyopathy and in three comparable control samples from accident victims as described for the monocrotaline-treated rats.

The two-dimensional analysis of myosin light chains from ventricles of patients in heart failure with idiopathic dilated cardiomyopathy showed only trace amounts of the additional light chain myosin, which were detectable exclusively in the subendocardial layers (Figure 11.5a). Mid-wall and subepicardium did not show such an additional atrial-like light chain 1. The picture was essentially the same as that observed in the control samples. Moreover, in the atria of patients with dilated cardiomyopathy, an additional light chain 2 of ventricular type was always present (Figure 11.5b). Such an additional ventricular light chain, which was identified by performing an immunoblot with anti-ventricular light chain 2 antibodies, never appeared in the control atria. This ventricular-like light chain myosin appearing in the atria seems to be the same isoform previously described in pressure or volume overloaded atria[70] and, like in hypertrophy, may have an adaptive significance.

The main finding of this study is that the additional atrial-like light chain myosin is nearly absent in subepicardial layers and mid-wall of patients with dilated cardiomyopathies. It is only faintly represented in the subendocardial layers, as well as in controls. These data apparently differ from those reported by Hirzel *et al.*[69] in a study carried out on endomyocardial biopsies from patients with dilated cardiomyopathies and various types of pressure or volume overload. These authors found that the atrial-like light chain is mainly expressed in the early stages of hypertrophy and of dilated cardiomyopathies in patients without significant changes in cardiac index

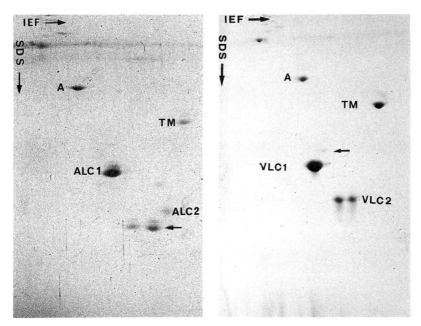

Figure 11.5 (*a*) Two-dimensional gel-electrophoresis of myosin light chains from left ventricle (subendocardial layer) of a patient with severe idiopathic cardiomyopathy. The arrow indicates the additional atrial-like light chain 1 which is barely discernible. ALC1 = atrial light chain 1; ALC2 = atrial light chain 2; IEF = first dimension carried out with isoelectrofocusing (migration according to electric charge); SDS = second dimension carried out in the presence of sodium dodecyl sulphate (migration according to molecular weight). (*b*) Two-dimensional gel electrophoresis of myosin light chains from left atrium of a patient with severe idiopathic cardiomyopathy. The arrow indicates the additional ventricular-like light chain 2. A = Actin; TM = tropomyosin; VLC1 = ventricular light chain 1; VCL2 = ventricular light chain 2

and in left ventricular end diastolic pressure. The changes we described are, on the contrary, obtained in patients in class IV of the New York grading system. It seems likely that, during ventricular failure, the myocardium loses the capability to express further the additional atrial-like light chain, which probably represents the fetal-type light chain 1. It is worth noting that our atrial samples still maintain the additional light chain of ventricular type despite the concomitant disappearance of the atrial-like myosin in ventricles. This fact probably reflects the lower stress which the atrial wall is subjected to and again suggests that the additional myosin light chains may play an adaptive role only in the early stage of overload.

The Ca^{2+}-activated ATP-ase activity of ventricular myosin in patients with cadiomyopathy showed a 60% reduction in comparison with controls (Table 11.3). The atrial activity is about twofold higher than the ventricular one in these patients, with a ratio similar to that described in the literature for normal hearts. A decrease in myofibrillar ATPase activity has been previously described in humans with cardiac hypertrophy and failure[71,72]. In other studies the Ca^{2+}-activated ATPase activity activated by calcium and assessed on purified myosins did not show any significant difference, at least between normal and hypertrophied, non-failing hearts[73,74]. The data here reported show that, in cardiac failure, Ca^{2+}-activated levels of ATPase in

Table 11.3 Myosin Ca^{2+}-activated ATPase activity (μmolPi/min/mg protein) in patients with idiopatic dilated cardiomyopathy and in normal subjects (mean $\pm$ SD)

	Normal subjects (n = 3)	Idiopathic dilated cardiomyopathy (n = 8)
Right atria	–	0.37 ± 0.07
Right ventricles	–	0.17 ± 0.02
Left atria	–	0.37 ± 0.04
Left ventricles	0.41 ± 0.09	0.15 ± 0.02

purified myosin are also reduced. Such a biochemical change could not be attributed to structural changes occurring in ventricular myosin heavy chains. Immunohistochemical studies indicate that the ventricular myocardium in humans possesses a low potential to shift toward the low-ATPase isoform of myosin, that is V$_3$[68]. Accordingly, on post-mortem material, no significant redistribution in ventricular isoenzymes was found in the hypertrophic myocardium in comparison with that from normal subjects[75].

Since, in the skeletal muscle, light chain 1 is involved in cross-bridging myosin to actin[76], it has been suggested that the change in myosin light chain composition can account for the reduction in ATPase activity[69]. In the present study we show that the fall in ATPase activity of myosin Ca^{2+}-activated ATPase activity occurring in failing heart is not paralleled by structural changes at the light chain level. There is still a missing link between alterations in biochemical and contractile properties of human ventricular myocardium and changes at molecular level of the contractile proteins. Whatever the mechanism leading to a fall in ATPase activity of ventricular myosin may be, this fall by itself implies a reduction in velocity of muscle shortening[77] and impending decompensation[57].

Beta-adrenergic responsiveness in cardiac hypertrophy and failure

The decreased inotropic function of the myocardium is the main alteration detectable in patients with congestive heart failure. In spite of the number of studies carried out both in humans and in animal models of heart failure, the pathophysiology of the failing myocyte is still unknown. One of the mechanisms that have been proposed to explain the reduced inotropism of the myocardial cells is a primary defect of the specialized component which modulates fluxes of calcium through the cell membrane[78]. Bristow *et al.* focused their attention on the beta-adrenergic cascade[79]. The beta-adrenoceptor, in coupling with its specific agonist, produces a stimulation of the adenylate-cyclase which in turn increases the intracellular concentration of cyclic AMP. Cyclic AMP phosphorylates the calcium-channel proteins and promotes influx of calcium. A direct effect of the beta-adrenoceptor, when complexed with the transducer guanine-nucleotide-binding protein (Gs), has also been shown on the sarcolemmal calcium channel[80].

A reduced sensitivity to beta-adrenoceptor stimulation has been reported in patients with heart failure. A decrease in adrenoceptor density in hearts from patients with chronic heart failure has been demonstrated in binding studies[79,81,82]. A decline in production of isoprenaline-stimulated cyclic AMP was also observed[79,82]. Contractile responses of isolated papillary muscles and trabecula from patients in heart failure to stimulation by beta-agonists were also markedly reduced[44,79]. This change in sensitivity may be an important factor contributing to the reduced reserve of contractile function in patients with heart failure. It has been suggested that an agonist-induced desensitization of beta-adrenoceptors occurs, due to increased exposure to catecholamines. It is known that prolonged exposure during life of animals to catecholamines decreases sensitivity to beta-agonists[83]. Treatment of cultured cardiac cells with isoprenaline also produced a reduction in beta-adrenoceptor density as well as adenylate cyclase activity[84] and contractile function stimulated by beta-agonists[85]. The mechanisms underlying the desensitization process include uncoupling of receptors from adenylate-cyclase activity, internalization and eventual loss of receptors. Patients with heart failure show raised levels of circulating catecholamines[86] and increased excretion of catecholamines[87]. Thomas and Marks[86] demonstrated a correlation between the degree of left ventricular dysfunction and levels of plasma norepinephrine.

Several lines of experimental evidence, however, appear to conflict with the theory of agonist-induced beta-adrenoceptor desensitization in heart failure. Work by Brown et al.[88] and Feldman et al.[44] suggests that the failing human heart shows reduced responsiveness not only to stimulation by beta-agonists but also to other inotropic agents acting through cyclic AMP, namely histamine and phosphodiesterase inhibitors. Work with cardiomyopathic hamsters had demonstrated an up-regulation of both β- and α_1-receptors. An increased inotropic response to norepinephrine accompanies heart failure in these animals.[89]. There are also methodological difficulties which often complicate the interpretation of data from human tissue. Although the patients in heart failure had not received catecholamines within the previous 24 hours, they might have been treated with diuretics, vasodilators, or digitalis, which could have affected the contraction of the isolated papillary muscle. Severely failing hearts are likely to have undergone hypertrophy which, in itself, may account for some reduction in density of beta-adrenoceptors. The presence of fibrotic tissue in the failing hearts may also have reduced the inotropic responsiveness of the papillary muscles.

We have investigated changes in the function of single cells in animal models of heart failure and agonist-induced desensitization, and compared them with alterations in human disease. In the rabbit with adriamycin-induced cardiomyopathy, a mild to moderate degree of failure occurs. The response of single ventricular myocytes isolated from the failing left ventricle to calcium and isoprenaline was studied. In these cells we detected a depressed maximum amplitude of contraction. This, once again, confirms the ability to detect depression of contractility in individual muscle cells from a failing heart. There was no evidence, however, of a specific beta-adrenoceptor desensitization. The isoprenaline-induced contraction was reduced to the same extent that of calcium, and the sensitivity to isoprenaline (concentration for half-maximal effect) was the same in normal and cardiomyopathic animals[39]. These results agree with findings on whole muscle from the hearts of adriamycin-treated animals[90]. In this model of failure, therefore, beta-adrenoceptor desensitization does not occur, despite raised catecholamine levels[90].

A question is whether in cardiac hypertrophy, which almost invariably precedes failure, a certain reduction of the inotropic responsiveness to adrenergic stimulation is present. Saragoca and Tarazi in two models of hypertension (spontaneously hypertensive rat and renovascular hypertensive rat[91,92], detected, both during life and in removed tissues, a decreased responsiveness to isoprenaline. Because the response to other inotropic stimuli, such as calcium and cardiac glycosides, was normal, this abnormality was related to a decreased myocardial beta-receptor density[93]. They also confirmed these data by radio-ligand experiments[94]. Fouad et al.[95], using renovascular hypertensive rats, also described an impaired inotropic response of the left ventricle to glucagon and vasoactive intestinal peptide. They suggested that left ventricular hypertrophy in such rats is not only dependent on a beta-receptor abnormality but extends to the adenylate-cyclase cascade. Other investigators reported that, in renal hypertension, the number of beta-receptors was either unchanged[96] or increased[97]. They thought this abnormality to be consistent with a reduction in the component of nucleotide regulatory protein of the adenylate-cyclase system. The data reported in the literature may sometimes appear conflicting. This could partly be due to the different experimental procedures used.

In the monocrotaline-treated rat, where ventricular hypertrophy and eventually failure occur, there was no decrease in maximum contraction amplitude with calcium or isoprenaline in either left or right ventricle of treated animals. Right ventricle cells from treated rats showed a two-fold increase in concentration of isoprenaline required for half-maximal effect compared with right ventricle cells from controls. There was no such shift in left ventricle cells. Plasma catecholamine levels were variable, but the urinary excretion of norepinephrine in the treated animals was significantly higher than that of controls. This model provides evidence against a role played by circulating catecholamines in desensitization, since these should affect left and right ventricles equally. Either local changes in catecholamines, or an interaction between hypertrophy and beta-adrenoceptor sensitivity as suggested above, may be responsible for the preferential loss of response in the right ventricular cells.

Though a diminished sensitivity to isoprenaline exists in these animals, the decrease is small if compared with those previously reported for human patients in heart failure[41]. This suggests that the mechanisms of cardiac adaptation in hypertrophy and failure may vary between species, and that animal models may have only a limited usefulness in determining the aetiology of human disease. We have, therefore, investigated the changes in beta-adrenoceptor sensitivity in isolated ventricular and atrial myocytes prepared from non-failing and failing human hearts. The patients and methods for cell isolation are as described above in the section 'Muscle Cell Characteristics'.

The loss of effectiveness of beta-adrenoceptor agonists on failing heart muscle could be detected at the level of the single atrial or ventricular mycocytes as a decrease in the maximum response to isoprenaline[98,99] The decrease in the maximum contraction attainable with isoprenaline does not represent a generalized defect in the contraction of the myocyte, since the maximum produced by calcium does not change with any indicator of heart failure (see above). In fact, the decline in the isoprenaline/calcium response ratio was more strongly related to the severity of disease than the isoprenaline maximum alone. For the left ventricle, ratios of one were only seen in donor hearts. Significant correlations were detected between the decrease in the ratio of isoprenaline to calcium in cells from the left ventricle and increasing severity of disease as defined by a number of criteria. These were the New York Heart Association class of symptoms of the patient (Figure 11.6; $p < 0.001$, $n = 15$ patients), left ventricular ejection fraction ($p < 0.01$, $n = 13$), left ventricular end diastolic pressure ($p < 0.02$, $n = 9$) and amount of diuretics prescribed ($p < 0.01$, $n = 15$). This was true for pooled ($n = $ patients) or non-pooled ($n = $ cells) data, and whether the results for patients who had been treated with beta-adrenoceptor agonist or antagonist drugs were included or excluded (unpublished observations). Comparison of the ratio of isoprenaline to calcium ratio between different classes of disease, rather than by severity, showed that there was little association of desensitization with one particular aetiology. Several groups have come to similar conclusions from studies of intact tissue. Depressed responses to isoprenaline have been seen in muscle strips from patients with ischaemic heart disease, mitral valve disease or idiopathic dilated cardiomyopathy [44,82,88,100].

Changes distal to the beta-adrenoceptor

To test the role of cyclic AMP production in beta-adrenoceptor subsensitivity, we have treated human atrial and ventricular myocytes with forskolin (which activates adenylate cyclase directly) and dibutyryl cyclic AMP (which penetrates the cell and mimics the effect of cyclic AMP). It is clear that the effect of both these agents are reduced at the same time as those of isoprenaline, indicating an alteration distal to the receptor (Figure 11.7). We have noticed that the concentration/response curve to isoprenaline can be limited in either of two ways. In one case the contraction amplitude stabilizes, and does not increase further with increasing concentrations of isoprenaline. In the second, the toxic effects of isoprenaline (prolonged after-contractions leading to merged beats, or arrythmias) prevent the contraction amplitude from rising more, despite the fact that the amplitude is well below the maximum attained with high calcium. In the first case, the phosphodiesterase inhibitor IBMX may increase the effect of isoprenaline until toxicity becomes evident at a higher amplitude. This implies a defect in cyclic AMP production in the cell. In the second case, neither forskolin nor dibutyryl cyclic AMP can produce a higher amplitude than isoprenaline, and IBMX does not enhance isoprenaline's action. This implies that, in this instance, the toxic effects of cyclic AMP are the limiting factor in

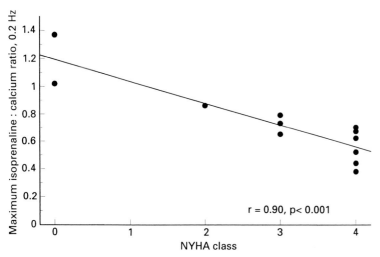

Figure 11.6 Left ventricular myocytes, results pooled for each patient. Dependence of contraction amplitude on New York Heart Association class of symptoms of patient/donor. Ratio of maximum isoprenaline to maximum calcium in the same cell

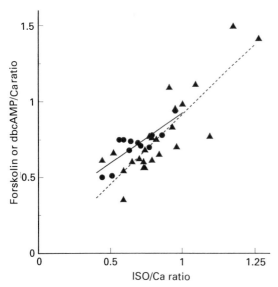

Figure 11.7 Correlation between the depression of the isoprenaline:calcium (ISO/CA) ratio for a ventricular myocyte and the forskolin (●——● , r = 0.69, p < 0.02) or dbcAMP (▲---▲ , r = 0.73, p < 0.001) response. Data from individual cells

the response. The results with dibutyryl cyclic AMP indicate that there is a defect unrelated to cyclic AMP production.

These findings are not incompatible with the hypothesis that desensitization is secondary to raised plasma catecholamines. Experiments on cultured neonatal rat myocytes suggest that exposure to noradrenaline initially produces a desensitization that appears functionally homologous for beta-adrenoceptor agonists[101] Longer treatment, however, gives a more complex pattern. We have performed similar experiments in adult rats by implanting mini-osmotic pumps subcutaneously, to give a continuous infusion of noradrenaline. Low doses of noradrenaline decreased the responses of myocytes isolated from the hearts of treated animals to isoprenaline, but the effects of forskolin or dibutyryl cyclic AMP were unaltered. Longer infusion with higher doses of noradrenaline reduced isoprenaline, forskolin and dibutyryl cyclic AMP responses in left ventricular cells, giving a profile of desensitization similar to that of the human myocytes from failing hearts. It is, therefore, possible for increases in plasma catecholamines to account for the changes in the adenylate cyclase cascade seen in failure. The differences reported by various authors in the pattern of change in heart failure could be due to the stage of the disease at which the study took place.

Interestingly, the response to catecholamine exposure was slower to develop in the right ventricles of the treated rats, even after the longer treatment with noradrenaline. The reduction in the beta-adrenoceptor and forskolin responses was smaller than in left, and the response to dibutyryl cyclic AMP was unaffected. We also had difficulty showing a correlation between severity of disease and depression of beta-adrenoceptor function in the right ventricle cells from the human subjects. We had attributed this to the fact that all the tissue from the right ventricle was obtained from explanted hearts, so that the majority of patients would have been in end-stage heart failure. Nevertheless, the possibility of a chamber-specific variation cannot be discounted. In eight transplant patients with ischaemic cardiomyopathy, cells were obtained from both right and left ventricle. There was a significant correlation between the ratio of isoprenaline to calcium in cells from the left and from the right ventricle. Right ventricular cells from these patients were slightly less desensitized than left; the regression line lying to the left of the line of identity. The ratio of isoprenaline to calcium in left ventricular myocytes was 0.64 ± 0.04, compared with 0.75 ± 0.04 in right ventricular cells ($n = 8$, $p < 0.01$, paired t-test, pooled data). The most striking difference between ventricles was seen in one patient with myocarditis, where the ratio of isoprenaline to calcium was depressed in two cells from the left ventricle (0.68) but close to unity in two cells from the right (1.18). These results are in agreement with those of Bristow *et al.*, who found evidence for a chamber-specific effect in studies on whole muscle taken from heart failure patients[79].

Summary

Our results have shown that animal models of hypertrophy and heart failure, although useful in some respects, must be applied with caution when making comparisons with human disease. The method of adaptation of the hearts of small mammals to increased load, through shifts in isozyme composition, is not necessarily mimicked by the human heart. The adaptation of the beta-adrenoceptor system, in particular, appears to be highly model dependent. Animal models have been helpful in validating the use of single isolated cardiac myocytes to make deductions about larger scale changes in failing hearts. Characterization of myocytes from failing human hearts have shown specific lesions in the beta-adrenoceptor system, which may result from profound changes in the way that cyclic AMP alters the calcium-handling of the cell. These alterations are consistent with an effect of raised catecholamine levels. The basic contractile characteristics of the cells, when maximally activated by high calcium, are not strongly related to the severity of failure, but more to the age of the patient.

Acknowledgements

The scientific contributions of Professor A. Burlina, Dr M. Zaninotto, Dr D. Piccolo and Dr M. Guardiano are acknowledged with gratitude. We are also grateful to Peter O'Gara, Mary Jones and Nicholas Hunt, who performed some of the experiments on human and animal myocytes.

References

1. Wikman-Coffelt, J., Parmley, W.W. and Mason, D.T. The cardiac hypertropy process: Analyses of factors determining pathological vs. physiological development. *Circ. Res.*, **45**, 697–707, 1979
2. Grossman, W. Cardiac hypertropy: Useful adaptation or pathological process? *Am. J. Med.*, **69**, 576–584, 1980
3. Bishop, S.P. and Altshuld, R.A. Increased glycolytic metabolism in cardiac hypertrophy and congestive failure. *Am. J. Physiol.*, **218**, 153–159, 1970
4. Revis, N.W., Thompson, R.Y. and Cameron, A.J.V. Lactate dehydrogenase isoenzymes in the human hypertropic heart. *Cardiovasc Res.*, **11**, 172–176, 1977

5. Anversa, P., Vitali-Mazza, L., Visioli, O. and Marchetti, G. Experimental cardiac hypertropy: A quantitative ultrastructural study in the compensatory stage. *J. Mol. Cell. Cardiol.*, **3**, 213–227, 1971

6. Goldstein, M.A., Sordahl, L.A. and Schwartz, A. Ultrastructural analysis of left ventricular hypertropy in rabbits. *J. Mol. Cell. Cardiol.*, **6**, 265–273, 1974

7. Page, E. and McAllister, L.P. Quantitative electron microscopic description of heart muscle cells. Application to normal, hypertropied and thyroxin-stimulated hearts. *Am. J. Cardiol.*, **31**, 172–181, 1973

8. Sordahl, L.A., McCollum, W.B., Wood, W.G. and Schwartz, A. Mitochondria and sarcoplasmic reticulum function in cardiac hypertropy and failure. *Am. J. Physiol.*, **224**, 497–502, 1973

9. Lindenmayer, G.E., Sordahl, L.A. and Schwartz, A. Reevaluation of oxidative phosphorylation in cardiac mitochondria from normal animals in heart failure. *Circ. Res.*, **23**, 439–450, 1968

10. Meerson, F.Z., Zaletayeva, T.A., Lagutchev, S.S. and Pshennikova, M.G. Structure and mass of mitochondria in the process of compensatory hyperfunction and hypertropy of the heart. *Exp. Cell. Res.*, **36**, 568–578, 1964

11. Ingwall, J.S. The hypertrophied myocardium accumulates the MB creatine-kinase isoenzyme. *Eur. Heart J.*, **5**, 124–139, 1984

12. Ingwall, J.S., Kramer, F. and Fifer, M.A. The creatine-kinase system in normal and diseased human myocardium. *N. Engl. J. Med.*, **313**, 1050–1054, 1985

13. Marchisino, M., Malvino, R. and Massaglia, A. Creatine-kinase forms in human skeletal and cardiac muscle. *Clin. Chim. Acta.*, **92**, 45–52, 1979

14. Sirageldin, E., Gercken, D., Harm, K. and Voight, K.D. The isoelectric focusing of creatine-kinase variants: The heterogeneity of creatine-kinase in human heart cytosol and mitochondria. *J. Clin. Chem. Clin. Biochem.*, **24**, 283–292, 1986

15. Bendz, R., Strom, S. and Olin, C. CK-MB in serum and heart and skeletal muscles in patients subjected to mitral valve replacement. *Eur. J. Cardiol.*, **12**, 25–39, 1980

16. Silven, C., Jansson, E. and Olin, C. Human myocardial and skeletal muscle enzyme activities: creatine-kinase and its isoenzyme MB as related to citrate synthetase and muscle fibre types. *Clin. Physiol.*, **3**, 461–468, 1983

17. Pauletto, P., Nascimben, L., Piccolo, D. *et al.* Ventricular myosin and creatine-kinase isoenzymes in hypertensive rats treated with captopril. *Hypertension;* **14**, 556–562, 1989

18. Younes, A., Schneider, J.M., Bergovic, J. and Swynghedauw, B. Redistribution of creatine-kinase isoenzymes in chronically overloaded myocardium. *Cardiovasc. Res.*, **19**, 15–19, 1984

19. Eppenberg, H.N., Dawson, D.M. and Kapplan, N.O. The comparative enzymology of creatine-kinase. Isolation and characterization from chicken and rabbit tissue. *J. Biol. Chem.*, **242**, 204–209, 1967

20. Szasz, G. and Gruber, W. Creatine-kinase in serum. Difference in substrate affinity among the isoenzymes. *Clin. Chem.*, **24**, 245–249, 1968

21. Ingwall, J., Kramer, F., Fifer, M.A. and Lorell, B. Changes in creatine-kinase isoenzyme distribution in hypertropied human myocardium. *Circulation*, **68**, III–65 (Abstract), 1983

22. Lowry, O.H., Rosenbrough, N.J., Farr, A.L. and Randall, R.J. Protein measurement with the Folin phenol reagent. *J. Biol. Chem.*, **193**, 265–270, 1951

23. Guidelines of the German Society for Clinical Chemistry. *Z. Klin. Chem. Biochem.*, **15**, 255–360, 1977

24. Haralambie, G. and Uy, J. Enzymes activities of human myocardium: creatine-kinase and hexose phosphate isomerase. *Clin. Cardiol.*, **3**, 192–196, 1980

25. Bittl, J.A. and Ingwall, J.S. Intracellular high-energy phosphate transfer in normal and hypertrophied myocardium. *Circulation*, **75**, 96–101, 1987

26. Schreiber, S.S., Oratz, M. and Rothschild, M.A. Protein synthesis in the overloaded mammalian heart. *Am. J. Physiol.*, **211**, 314–318, 1966

27. Schreiber, S.S., Oratz, M., Rothschild, M.A. and Reff, F. The effect of hydrostatic pressure on isolated cardiac nuclei. Stimulation of RNA II polymerase activity. *Cardiovasc. Res.*, **12**, 265–268, 1978

28. Morgan, H.E., Bhua, B.H.L., Siehl, D., *et al.*, Factors controlling the efficiency of protein synthesis in the heart. In *Myocardial Hypertropy and Failure* (ed N.R. Alpert), Raven Press, New York, pp. 425–431, 1983

29. Caufield, J.B. and Borg, T.K. The collagen network of the heart. *Lab. Invest.*, **40**, 364, 1979

30. Turto, H. and Lindy, S. Collagen metabolism of the rat heart during experimental cardiac hypertropy and the effect of digitonin treatment. *Adv. Cardiol.*, **18**, 41, 1976

31. Caufield, J.B. Morphologic alterations of the collagen matrix with cardiac hypertropy. In *Myocardial Hypertropy and Failure* (ed N.R. Alpert), Raven Press, New York, pp. 167–175, 1983

32. Weber, K.T., Janicki, J.S., Shroff, S. and Pearlman, E.S. Shape and structure of the normal and failing human heart. In *Myocardial Hypertropy and Failure* (ed N.R. Alpert), Raven Press, New York, pp. 85–102, 1983

33. Bing, O.H., Matsushito, S., Fanburg, B.L. and Levine, H.J. Mechanical properties of rat cardiac muscle during experimental hypertropy. *Circ. Res.*, **28**, 234–239, 1971

34. Weber, K.T., Janicki, J.S., Pick, R. and Abrahams, C. Collagen in the hypertrophied, pressure-overloaded myocardium. *Circulation*, **75(I)**, 1–40, 1987

35. Weber, K.T., Janicki, J.S., Shroff, S. *et al.* Collagen remodeling of the pressure-overloaded, hypertrophied nonhuman primate myocardium. *Circ. Res.*, **62**, 757–765, 1988

36. Harding, S.E., Vescovo, G., Kirby, M., *et al.* Contractile responses of isolated rat and rabbit myocytes to isoproterenol and calcium. *J. Mol. Cell. Cardiol.*, **20**, 635–647, 1988

37. Harding, S.E., Vescovo, G., Jones, S.M., *et al.* Morphological and functional characteristics of myocytes isolated from human left ventricular aneurysms. *J. Pathol.*, **1590**, 191–196, 1989

38. Harding, S.E., O'Gara, P., Jones, S.M., *et al.* Species dependence of contraction velocity in single isolated cardiac myocytes. *Cardioscience*, **10**, 49–53, 1990

39. Jones, S.M., Kirby, M.S., Harding, S.E., *et al.* Adriamycin cardiomyopathy in the rabbit: alterations in contractile proteins and myocyte function. *Cardiovasc. Res.*, (in press), 1990

40. Vescovo, G., Harding, S.E., Jones, S.M., *et al.* Comparison between isomyosin pattern and contractility of right ventricular myocytes isolated from rats with right cardiac hypertrophy. *Basic Res. Cardiol.*, **84**, 536–543, 1989

41. Vescovo, G., Jones, S.M., Harding, S.E. and Poole-Wilson, P.A. Isoproterenol sensitivity of isolated cardiac myocytes from rats with monocrotaline-induced right-sided hypertrophy and heart failure. *J. Mol. Cell Cardiol.*, **21**, 1047–1061, 1989

42. Jones, S.M., Gurden, J., Harding, S.E. and Poole-Wilson, P.A. Beta-adrenoceptor desensitisation in papillary muscles and myocytes from the hearts of isoprenaline-treated rabbits. *J. Mol. Cell Cardiol.*, **21 Suppl II**, 199 (Abstract), 1989

43. Ginsburg, R., Esserman, L.J. and Bristow, M.R. Myocardial performance and extracellular ionised calcium in a severely failing human heart. *Ann. Intern. Med.*, **98**, 603–606, 1983

44. Feldman, M.D., Copelas, B.S., Gwathmey, J.K., *et al.* Deficient production of cyclic AMP: pharmacologic evidence of an important cause of contractile dysfunction in patients with end-stage failure. *Circulation*, **2**, 331–339, 1987

45. Bohm, M., Beukelmann, D., Brown, L., *et al.* Reduction of beta-adrenoceptor density and evaluation of positive inotropic responses in isolated diseased human myocardium. *Eur. Heart J.*, **9**, 844–852, 1988

46. Gwathmey, J.K., Copelas, L., MacKinnon, R., *et al.* Abnormal calcium handling in myocardium from patients with end-stage heart failure. *Circ. Res.*, **61**, 70–76, 1987

47. Schwartz, K., De La Bastie, D., Bouveret, P. and Oliviero, P. Alpha-skeletal muscle actin mRNA's accumulate in hypertropied adult rat hearts. *Circ. Res.*, **59**, 551–555, 1986

48. Leger, J., Klotz, C. and Leger, J.J. Cardiac myosin heavy chains and tropomyosin in mechanical heart overloading and aging. In *Myocardial Hypertropy and Failure*, (ed N.R. Alpert), Raven Press, New York, pp. 385–392, 1983

49. Schwartz, K., Lecarpentier, Y. and Martin, J.L. Myosin isoenzymic distribution correlates with speed of muscle shortening. *J. Mol. Cell Cardiol.*, **13**, 1071–1075, 1981

50. Kissling, G., Rupp, H., Malloy, L. and Jacob, R. Alteration in cardiac oxygen consumption under chronic pressure overload: significance of the isoenzyme pattern of myosin. *Basic Res. Cardiol.*, **77**, 225–269, 1982

51. Hoh, J.F., McGrath, P.A. and Hale, P.T. Electrophoretic analysis of multiple forms of rat cardiac myosin: Effects of hypophysectomy and thyroxine replacement. *J. Mol. Cell Cardiol.*, **10**, 1053–1076, 1978

52. Lompre, A.M., Mercadier, J.J. and Wisnewsky, C. Species and age dependent changes in the relative amounts of cardiac myosin isoenzymes in mammals. *Dev. Biol.*, **84**, 286–290, 1981

53. Gorza, L., Pauletto, P., Pessina, A.C., *et al.* Isomyosin redistribution in normal and hypertrophic rat ventricular myocardium: an immunohistochemial study. *Circ. Res.*, **49**, 1003–1009, 1981

54. Pauletto, P., Vescovo, G., Scannapieco, G., *et al.* Changes in rat ventricular isomyosins with regression of cardiac hypertrophy. *Hypertension*, **8**, 1143–1148, 1986

55. Alpert N.R. and Mulieri, L.A. Increased economy of isometric force generation in compensated cardiac hypertropy induced by pulmonary artery constriction in the rabbit: a characterization of heat liberation in normal hypertropied right ventricular papillary muscle. *Circ. Res.*, **77**, 225–269, 1982

56. Morano, I., Gagelmann, M., Arner, A. and Ganten, U. Myosin isoenzymes of vascular smooth and

cardiac muscle in the spontaneously hypertensive and normotensive male and female rat: a comparative study. *Circ. Res.*, **59**, 456–462, 1986

57. Swynghedauw, B., Schwartz, K. and Apstein, C.S. Decreased contractility after myocardial hypertrophy: cardiac failure or successful adaptation? *Am. J. Cardiol.*, **54**, 437–440, 1984

58. Swynghedauw, B. Moalic, J.M. and Lecarpentier, Y. Adaptive changes of contractile proteins in chronic cardiac overloading: structure and rate of synthesis. In *Myocardial Hypertropy and Failure* (ed. N.R. Alpert), Raven Press, New York, pp. 465–476, 1983

59. Dillman, W.H. Hormonal influences on cardiac myosin ATPase activity and myosin isoenzymes distribution. *Mol. Cell Endocrinol.*, **34**, 169–181, 1984

60. Malhotra, A. Schaible, T. and Scheuer, J. Effect of testosterone on cardiac myosin in rats. *J. Mol. Cell Cardiol.*, **15 (Suppl. 1)**, 316, 1983

61. Sen, S. and Young, D.R. Role of sodium in modulation of myocardial hypertropy in renal hypertensive rats. *Hypertension*, **8**, 918–924, 1986

62. Steter, FA., Faris, R., Balogh, J. and Somogyi, E. Changes in myosin isoenzyme distribution induced by low doses of isoproterenol. *Arch. Int. Pharmacodyn.*, **260**, 159–164, 1982

63. Rupp, H. The adaptive changes in isoenzymes pattern of myosin from hypertrophied rat myocardium as a result of pressure overload and physical training. *Basic Res. Cardiol.*, **76**, 79–88, 1981

64. Dalla Libera, L., Pauletto, P., Angelini, A., *et al.* Biochemical characterization of ventricular myosin from spontaneously hypertensive turkeys. *J. Mol. Cell Cardiol.*, **17**, 1019–1022, 1985

65. Balint, M., Streter, F.A., Wolf, J., *et al.* The substructure of heavy meromyosin. *J. Biol. Chem.*, **250**, 6168–6177, 1975

66. Lanzetta, P.A., Alvarez, L.J., Reinach, P.S. and Candia, O.A. An improved assay for nanomole amounts of inorganic phosphate. *Anal. Biochem.*, **100**, 95–98, 1979

67. O'Farrell, P.H. High resolution two-dimensional electrophoresis of proteins. *J. Biol. Chem.*, **250**, 4007–4010, 1975

68. Schiaffino, S., Gorza, L., Sartore, S. and Valfre, C. Adaptative changes in cardiac isomyosins as visualised by immunofluorescence. In *Cardiac Adaption to Hemodynamic Overload, Training and Stress* (eds R. Jacob, R.W. Gulch and G. Kissling), Steinkoppf Verlag: Damstadt, pp. 101–103, 1983

69. Hirzel, H.O., Tuchschmid, C.R. and Schneider, J. Relationship between myosin isoenzymes composition hemodynamics and myocardial structure in various forms of human cardiac hypertrophy. *Circ. Res.*, **57**, 729–740, 1985

70. Cummings, P. Transition in human atrial and ventricular myosin light chain isoenzymes in response to cardiac pressure-overload induced hypertropy. *Biochem. J.*, **205**, 195–204, 1982

71. Leclerq, J.F. and Swynghedauw, B. Myofibrillar ATPase, DNA and hydroxyproline content of human hypertrophied heart. *Eur. J. Clin. Invest.*, **6**, 27–33, 1976

72. Swynghedauw, B., Schwartz, K. and Leger, J.J. Cardiac myosin. Phylogenic and pathologic changes. *Basic Res. Cardiol.*, **72**, 254–260, 1977

73. Schier, J.J. and Aldestein, R.S. Structural and enzymatic comparison of human cardiac muscle myosin isolated from infants, adults and patients with hypertrophic cardiomyopathy. *J. Clin. Invest.*, **69**, 816–825, 1982

74. Mercadier, J.J., Bouveret, P., Gorza, L. and Schiaffino, S. Myosin isoenzymes in normal and hypertrophied human ventricular myocardium. *Circ. Res.*, **53**, 52–62, 1983

75. Gorza, L., Mercadier, J.J., Schwartz, K. and Thornell, L.E. Myosin types in the human heart. An immunofluorescence study of normal and hypertrophied atrial and ventricular myocardium. *Circ. Res.*, **54**, 694–702, 1984

76. Yamamoto, K. and Sekine, T. Interaction of alkali light chain-1 with actin: Effect of ionic strength on the cross-linking of alkali light chain-1 with actin. *J. Biochem. (Tokyo)*, **94**, 2075–2078, 1983

77. Barany, M. ATPase activity of myosin correlated with speed of muscle shortening. *J. Gen. Physiol.*, **50**, 197–202, 1967

78. Braunwald, E., Ross, J.Jr. and Sonnenblick, E.H. *Mechanism of Contraction of the Normal and Failing Heart*, Little Brown: Boston, p. 309. 1970

79. Bristow, M.R., Ginsburg, R., Minobe, B.S. and Cubicciotti, R.S. Decreased catecholamine sensitivity and beta-receptor density in failing human heart. *N. Engl. J. Med.*, **30**, 205–211, 1982

80. Yatani, A., Imoto, Y., Codina, J., *et al.* The stimulatory G protein of adenylyl cyclase. Gs, also stimulates dihydropyridine-sensitive Ca^{2+} channels. Evidence for direct regulation independent of phosphorylation by cAMP-dependent protein kinase or stimulation by a dihydropyridine agonist. *J. Biol. Chem.*, **263**, 9887–9895, 1988

81. Bristow, M.R., Ginsburg, R., Means, V. and Fowler, M. Beta1- and beta-adrenergic-receptor subpopulations in non-failing and failing human ventricular myocardium: Coupling of both

receptor subtypes to muscle contraction and selective beta1-receptor down regulation in heart failure. *Circ. Res.*, **59**, 297–309, 1986

82. Fowler, M.B., Laser, J.A., Hopkins, G.L. and Minobe, W. Assessment of the α-adrenergic receptor pathway in the intact failing human heart: progressive receptor down-regulation and subsensitivity to agonist response. *Circulation*, **74**, 1290–1302, 1986

83. Change, H.Y., Klein, R.M. and Kunos, G. Selective desensitisation of cardiac beta-adrenoceptors by prolonged in vivo infusion of catecholamines in rats. *J. Pharmacol. Exp. Ther.*, **221**, 784–789, 1981

84. Bobik, A., Campbell, J.H., Carson, V. and Campbell, G.R. Mechanism of isoprenaline induced refractoriness of the beta-adrenoceptor-adenylate cyclase system in chick embryo cardiac cells. *J. Cardiovasc. Pharmacol.*, **3**, 541–553, 1981

85. Marsh, J.D. and Roberts. D.J. Adenylate cyclase regulation in intact cultured myocardial cells. *Am. J. Physiol.*, **252**, C47–C54, 1987

86. Thomas, J.A. and Marks, B.H. Plasma norepinephrine in congestive heart failure. *Am. J. Cardiol.*, **41**, 233–243, 1978

87. Chidsey, L.A., Braunwald, E. and Morrow, E.G. Catecholamine excretion and cardiac stores of norephinephrine in congestive heart failure. *Am. J. Med.*, **39**, 442–451, 1965

88. Brown, L., Lorenz, B. and Erdmann, E. Reduced positive inotropic effects in diseased human ventricular myocardium. *Cardiovasc. Res.*, **20**, 516–520, 1986

89. Karliner, J.S., Alabaster, C. and Stephens, H. Enhanced noradrenaline response in cadiomyopathic hamsters: possible relation to changes in adrenoceptors studied by radioligand binding. *Cardiovasc. Res,*, **15**, 296–304, 1981

90. Woodcock, E.A., Arnolda, L. and McGrath, B.P. Ventricular beta-adrenoceptors in adriamycin-induced cardiomyopathy in the rabbit. *J. Mol. Cell Cardiol.*, **20**, 771–777, 1988

91. Saragoca, M. and Tarazi, R.C. Impaired cardiac contractile response to isoproterenol in the spontaneously hypertensive rat. *Hypertension*, **3**, 380–385, 1981

92. Saragoca, M. and Tarazi, R.C. Left ventricular hypertropy in rats with renovascular hypertension. Alterations in cardiac function and adrenergic responses. *Hypertension*, **3**, 171–176, 1981

93. Ayobe, M.H. and Tarazi, R.C. Beta-receptors and contractile reserve in left ventricular hypertrophy. *Hypertension*, **5 (Suppl. 1)**, 192–197, 1983

94. Ayobe, M.H. and Tarazi, R.C. Reversal of changes in myocardial beta-receptors and inotropic responsiveness with regression of cardiac hypertropy in Renal Hypertensive Rats (RHR). *Circ. Res.*, **54**, 125–134, 1983

95. Fouad, F.M., Shimamatsu, K., Said, S.I. and Tarazi, R.C. Inotropic responsiveness in hypertensive left ventricular hypertrophy: Impaired inotropic response to glucagon and vasoactive intestinal peptide in renal hypertensive rats. *J. Cardiovasc. Pharmacol.*, **8**, 398–405, 1986

96. Gicchetti, A., Clark, T.L. and Berti, F. Subsensitivity of cardiac beta-adrenoceptors in renal hypertensive rats. *J. Cardiovasc. Pharmacol.*, **1**, 467–471, 1979

97. Kumano, K., Upsher, M.E. and Khairallah, P.A. Beta adrenergic receptor response coupling in hypertrophied hearts. *Hypertension*, **(Suppl. 1)**, 175, 1983

98. Harding, S.E., Jones, S.M., Vescovo, G. and Poole-Wilson, P.A. Response of human isolated atrial myocytes to forskolin and isoprenaline; relation to NYHA class. *Eur. Heart J.*, **11**, 1298 (Abstract), 1990

99. Harding, S.E., Jones, S.M., Vescovo, G., *et al.* Beta-adrenoceptor desensitisation in single ventricular cells isolated from failing human hearts. *Circulation*, **80(4)**, 1748 (Abstract), 1989

100. Bohm, M., Diet, F., Feiler, G., *et al.* Subsensitivity of the failing human heart to isoprenaline and milrinone is related to beta-adrenoceptor downregulation. *J. Cardiovasc. Pharmacol.*, **12**, 726–732, 1988

101. Reithmann, C. and Werdan, K. Homologous vs. heterologous desensitization of the adenylate cyclase system in heart cells. *Eur. J. Pharmacol.*, **154**, 99–104, 1988

12

The management of severe heart failure: Assessment, drug therapy, circulatory support, transplantation and rehabilitation

Nicholas Banner and Magdi Yacoub

Introduction

Important advances have been made in the management of heart failure during the last decade. It has now been established that medical therapy can not only relieve symptoms but also improve survival in patients with moderate to severe heart failure[1,2]. Cardiac transplantation has become a highly effective treatment for end-stage heart failure[3,4]. Other methods of treatment, including the use of mechanical circulatory support as a 'bridge' to transplantation[5] and the use of the automatic implantable cardioverter–defibrillator[6], are now being investigated.

Cardiac transplantation has, none the less, created new clinical problems, including the management of cardiac rejection and of opportunistic infections, together with those of rehabilitation after transplantation. The prevention and management of other complications (including cyclosporin nephrotoxicity, transplant hypertension and coronary arterial disease in the transplanted heart) are now becoming important issues[3]. The improved results of transplantation have resulted in an increase in referrals of patients, such that the number of patients who could potentially benefit from transplantation now exceeds the supply of donor organs[7]. The growing waiting list has highlighted the problems of management prior to transplantation. The cardiologist must attempt to control the patient's symptoms and ensure that his general condition will enable him to benefit from a transplant if it becomes possible.

This article reviews some of the recent developments in the management of severe heart failure and the role of heart transplantation, with particular reference to the experience obtained at our own centre (Table 12.1, Figure 12.1).

Assessment of the patient with severe heart failure

The goals of management of heart failure are to relieve symptoms, improve exercise capacity, enhance quality of life, extend survival and select patients appropriately for transplantation.

Clinical assessment and echocardiographic measurement of left ventricular dimensions and fractional shortening, or ejection fraction, will give an initial guide to the severity of ventricular impairment and prognosis[8,9]. Exacerbating factors, such as anaemia or infection, should be identified and treated. Drug therapy should be reviewed and adjusted. Once the patient is in a stable clinical condition, an assessment can be made of the aetiology of the heart failure and the suitability of the

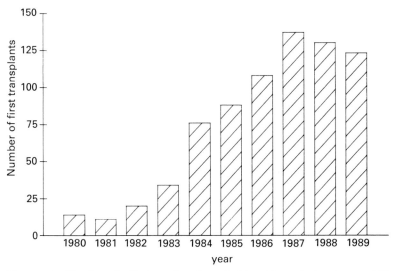

Figure 12.1 Number of patients undergoing a first heart transplant each year at Harefield and its associated hospitals. There was a rapid increase in the number of procedures performed as a result of the improved survival obtained after the introduction of cyclosporin in 1982. Transplantation is currently limited by the supply of suitable donor organs

patient for transplantation. It is best to consider the possibility of transplantation at an early stage because of the unpredictable nature of heart failure. The objective is to avoid, whenever possible, having to decide on the suitability for transplantation, or mechnical circulatory support, of a patient who has not been fully evaluated and who is now in an unstable, critically ill, condition. Patients who undergo emergency transplantation, without a period of preoperative counselling, experience more difficulty in adjusting psychologically afterwards. When investigational procedures (such as 'bridging' a deteriorating patient to transplantation with a ventricular assist

Table 12.1 Total experience with cardiopulmonary transplantation at Harefield Hospital and the National Heart and Lung Institute. Number of patients receiving each type of transplant at their first operation between January 1980 and September 1990. In addition, 54 patients have undergone a second transplant

Type of organ transplant	Number
Orthotopic heart	776
Heterotopic heart	41
Heart and kidney	1
Heart and liver	1
Combined heart–lung	278
Heart–lung and liver	3
Single lung	61
Double lung (en bloc)	3
Bilateral 'single' lung	3
Total	1167

device) are a possibility, this is best discussed with the patient while he is in a stable condition.

The principal indication for cardiac transplantation is heart failure that is so severe that it cannot be treated by other means; in other words, advanced heart failure due to ventricular dysfunction. The most common conditions leading to transplantation in our unit are end-stage ischaemic cardiomyopathy (53%) and idiopathic dilated cardiomyopathy (40%)[3]. Other indications include specific diseases of heart muscle, congenital heart disease with poor left ventricular function, valvar heart disease with poor left ventricular function (usually after a previous replacement of a valve) and the occasional patient with an unresectable cardiac tumour[10].

The patient must be able psychologically to cope with transplantation and to comply with the intensive follow-up required postoperatively, together with the need for life-long immunosuppression. This requires careful education and counselling during the process of assessment. In our experience, it is unusual to have to refuse transplantation because of psychological or social factors. Many psychological problems are related to the severity of the physical illness and resolve after transplantation. A history of depression, psychosis or substance abuse, however, requires a detailed psychiatric evaluation.

The introduction of cyclosporin as an immunosuppressive agent has been associated with an improvement in the results of transplantation[11]. It has also allowed us to extend the range of patients considered for transplantation. In particular, it has enabled transplants to be performed in children while avoiding the adverse effects of long-term steroid therapy on growth[12].

A variety of systemic conditions can increase the risks of transplantation and must be considered on an individual basis (Table 12.2)[3,13]. Any other condition that seriously limits the life expectancy of the patient normally precludes transplantation. Chronic infections may be exacerbated by immunosuppression, and patients previously treated for tuberculosis require chemoprophylaxis after transplantation. Patients who are positive for hepatitis B surface antigen, or have antibodies for the human immunodeficiency virus, are considered unsuitable for transplantation.

Age is not, in itself, a barrier to transplantation. We have successfully transplanted patients up to 69 years of age[19]. The limited supply of donor organs and the large number of younger patients requiring transplantation, none the less, must limit transplantation in those aged over 60 years. This problem can be ameliorated, to some extent, by public education and extending the criteria used for accepting donor organs[20].

It is important to establish the aetiology of the ventricular damage. The diagnosis of ischaemic heart disease should prompt an evaluation of the underlying risk factors. Patients who smoke must be encouraged to stop. Abnormalities in lipid metabolism are common in this group and require treatment because they can contribute to the subsequent development of coronary arterial disease in the transplanted heart[21,22].

Revascularization may be an option in some patients with heart failure due to ischaemic heart disease. Coronary bypass surgery will reduce the risk of further infarction. In combination with medical therapy and aneurysmectomy, if appropriate, it may result in a significant improvement in the condition of the patient. When ventricular damage is severe, however, the key issue is whether some of the dysfunction is due to 'stunned' or 'hibernating' myocardium and is potentially reversible with revascularization[23]. Several functional scanning techniques have been used in an attempt to predict reversibility with revascularization. These include re-injection of thallium after stress-redistribution thallium imaging[24] and positron

Table 12.2 Factors complicating cardiac transplantation

Condition	Comments
Renal failure	See text. Intrinsic renal disease can be treated by combined heart/kidney transplant
Pulmonary hypertension	See text
Systemic hypertension	Rarely severe in end-stage heart failure. Does not increase post transplant hypertension[14]
Pulmonary embolism/ infarction	Danger of pulmonary infarct becoming abscess with immunosuppression. Ideally allow to heal. Urgent transplant increases risk[15]
Peptic ulcer disease	Risk of perioperative re-activation and gastrointestinal haemorrhage. Document endoscopic healing. Prophylactic ranitidine with steroids
Diabetes	Avoid steroid immunosuppression. Patients with nephropathy, retinopathy or active infection unsuitable[16]
Cerebrovascular disease	Risk of perioperative stroke. Existing neurological deficit could compromise rehabilitation
Peripheral vascular disease	Not a contraindication unless severe. Complicates cardiac catheterization/IABP insertion. May influence rehabilitation. Steroids may acclerate disease
Psychiatric disorders	Important because of potential effect on compliance and rehabilitation. Assessment difficult in severely ill patients. Formal evaluation of those with history of depression, psychosis or substance-abuse
Epilepsy	Cyclosporin can cause post-operative convulsions. Major drug interactions between Cyclosporin and many anticonvulsants[17]
Obstructive airways disease	Common in smokers with IHD. Full respiratory assessment required. In severe cases consider combined heart–lung transplant
Liver disease	Intrinsic liver disease may limit life expectancy. Clotting abnormalities complicate surgery and drug metabolism altered. Combined transplant might be indicated
Systemic malignancy	Immunosuppression may reactivate/accelerate disease. Patients with high probability of 'cure' may benefit from transplant (e.g. adriamycin cardiomyopathy after lymphoma)[18]
Infection	Active infections should normally be treated before transplant. Bacterial infections easier to manage in absence of steroids. Chronic infections may reactivate – see text

emission tomography with a combination of nitrogen-13-ammonia and fluorine-18-deoxyglucose[25]. The utility of such investigations in the population of potential transplant candidates has not, however, been investigated.

We have performed revascularization with, or without, aneurysmectomy combined with heterotopic heart transplantation in 28 patients with severe heart failure due to ischaemic heart disease. This procedure has resulted in a 1-year survival rate of 79%. Functional status and rehabilitation has been satisfactory, with only one patient having recurrent angina. In most cases, the recipient's own heart has continued to contribute to the overall cardiac output, although in some cases there has been a progressive deterioration. It has been difficult to assess the impact of the reconstructive surgery on the function of the native heart because of the altered loading conditions due to the native and transplanted hearts functioning in parallel (Ridley *et al.*, unpublished observations).

When coronary angiography reveals normal arteries, or disease that is insufficient to explain the ventricular damage, myocardial biopsies are required. In cases of apparent idiopathic dilated cardiomyopathy, the question of excess intake of alcohol should be considered. Some specific diseases of heart muscle can recur after transplantation[26–28]. The explanted heart should be submitted for pathological examination at the time of transplantation.

When transplantation appears to be a therapeutic option, the pulmonary vascular resistance should be measured by right heart catheterization. An increased resistance is a recognized risk factor for cardiac transplantation because the normal right ventricle of the transplanted heart may fail postoperatively[13]. This is a particular problem in longstanding left ventricular failure. A high resistance can often be reduced by vasodilator therapy and is then usually considered benign. A variety of techniques have been used to deal with an elevated pulmonary vascular resistance, including using the heart of a larger donor, heterotopic transplantation, and heart–lung transplantation[3]. Our current approach to this problem is to transplant the heart from a suitable recipient of heart–lung transplantation (such as a patient requiring transplantation for respiratory failure secondary to cystic fibrosis) which has some pre-existing right ventricular hypertrophy – the 'Domino' transplant[29].

Renal function is of crucial importance. The mainstay of post-transplant immuno-suppression is cyclosporin, which is nephrotoxic[17,30]. Pre-existing renal dysfunction increases the risk of postoperative renal failure. In addition to the problems associated with renal failure and its treatment, this will make it difficult to use cyclosporin effectively and will increase the risk of cardiac rejection. The substitution of other, less specific, immunosuppressive agents will increase the incidence of infectious complications. Thus attempting to maintain good renal function is a major goal of the management of heart failure prior to transplantation. Impaired renal function may clearly be secondary to heart failure if the deterioration accompanied a worsening haemodynamic state, or if there is an improvement with appropriate cardiac therapy. In other circumstances, the possibility of intrinsic renal disease must be considered and further investigations conducted in consultation with a nephrologist. Radiographic or ultrasound evidence of contracted kidneys or abnormal urinary sediment on microscopy are often clues to an intrinsic renal problem.

Once a patient has been accepted for transplantation, a decision must be made about priority on the waiting list. This depends on both the severity of the current condition of the patient and the estimation of prognosis with medical therapy (see below).

Donor–recipient matching

Additional information is required to match the transplant candidate to organs from the potential donor. Matching of the size is done on the basis of height and weight. A discrepancy of up to 20% is usually considered acceptable. Patients with an increased pulmonary vascular resistance have special requirements and may require a larger donor or a 'Domino' transplant. Compatibility in terms of ABO blood grouping is considered essential. Recipients who have a positive lymphocytotoxic antibody screen (usually as a result of previous blood transfusion or pregnancy) will require a prospective cross-match against donor lymphocytes. We have found that, although a positive cross-match does not always lead to hyperacute rejection of the heart, it is associated with a reduced survival[31]. Although it is not possible routinely to perform matching for human leucocyte antigens in heart transplantation, all potential recipients undergo full tissue typing. Retrospective analysis has shown that partial matching, particularly at the HLA-DR locus, is associated with improved survival[32]. If two clinically stable patients, with a similar priority, are suitable for a particular donor heart, the candidate with a partial match at the DR locus should be favoured.

Cytomegalovirus antibody status should be determined. Candidates without antibodies to the virus should, whenever possible, receive an organ from a donor who is also antibody negative, and receive blood products which have been screened for antibodies. This reduces the risk of cytomegalovirus pneumonitis after transplantation[33].

The prognosis of heart failure

Several studies have examined variables that are associated with a poor survival in heart failure. These have confirmed the generally poor prognosis of advanced ventricular failure. One group has reported a high mortality in patients that they had considered 'too well' for transplantation – with a 1-year survival of only 46% without transplantation[34]. A variety of factors have been described as predictors of an increased mortality. These include a low ejection fraction[35–37], low peak uptake of oxygen during exercise[35], elevated circulating levels of noradrenaline[35], increased dimensions of the left ventricle[36], worse functional class[38,39], increased left ventricular filling pressure (end-diastolic or pulmonary wedge)[36,37,40], low cardiac output or stroke volume at rest[40]. All these factors are clearly related to the degree of ventricular dysfunction and its consequences. The relationship of ventricular arrhythmias to prognosis is controversial and is discussed below.

There are numerous difficulties in applying the results of such surveys in clinical practice. Most studies have looked for variables that are statistically associated with survival rather than attempting to produce a quantitative model predicting survival. Since most of the variables measured are correlated with one another, the parameters estimated in such a model would be unstable and highly dependent on the data used to derive them. No study has attempted to validate a survival model on a second set of patients. Step-wise regression procedures have been used to select 'independent' prognostic factors but, in the presence of multicollinearity, the variables selected will also be unstable[41]. This may account for some of the differences in the results of the various studies. The problem is compounded by the different measurements selected by various authors. A recent study has tried to overcome some of the problems by selecting three variables which were weakly correlated with each other: the level of noradrenaline level at rest, the left ventricular ejection fraction, and the peak uptake of oxygen during exercise[35]. All three variables appeared to contribute additional prognostic information.

Most studies have not focused specifically on patients suitable for transplantation. The spread of measurements in such a group is generally low. For example, ejection fraction has been found to be of prognostic significance in a wide range of patients, from those who have suffered a first myocardial infarction[42] to those with established heart failure[35–37]. In the population of candidates for transplantation, however, most patients have ejection fractions clustered around 15–20%, making it impossible to discriminate reliably between individuals.

An important question is whether a change in clinical status during follow-up can be used to indicate prognosis. Since many deaths related to heart failure are sudden[43], this approach has serious limitations. One study found that, in patients with idiopathic dilated cardiomyopathy, about half the patients who died had a clinically recognized deterioration before death[36]. Long-term survivors often had a stable or improved functional capacity. It was observed that those who survived for more than 5 years after diagnosis had a very low rate of death, suggesting that a subgroup of these patients have stable and non-progressive disease[36].

There is limited information about the influence of drug-induced changes on the relationships to prognosis of symptoms and haemodynamic status. Vasodilator therapy can improve ejection fraction, and it has been suggested that changes in ejection fraction might be used as a surrogate measure for survival in future drug studies, although this relationship has not been clearly established[44].

A pragmatic approach is to monitor several variables which are not strongly correlated, such as echocardiographic ejection fraction and exercise capacity (peak oxygen uptake) and levels of noradrenaline, together with the symptomatic status of the patient. The interpretation of the changes must be tempered by an appreciation of the limited reproducibility of such measurements[45]. Deterioration is a series cause for concern. Stability or improvement, in contrast, may provide some degree of reassurance, although it may not indicate a low risk of sudden death[46]. Periodic catheterization of the right heart, to determine pulmonary vascular resistance for possible transplantation, can provide further information about left-sided filling pressures which cannot reliably be assessed clinically in patients with chronic heart failure[47].

A different approach to evaluating the degree of ventricular failure is to stress the ventricle pharmacologically. One study investigated the response to the calcium antagonist nifedipine[48]. Haemodynamic deterioration after a single dose was associated with worse subsequent survival. Some of the patients, however, experienced a cardiovascular collapse during the test. The authors concluded that such methods are potentially dangerous in patients with severe heart failure. A more promising technique may be to examine the acute response of cardiac power output to inotropic stimulation[49]. Patients with low maximum cardiac power output have a worse prognosis. It has not been established how this index relates to other measures of ventricular performance and prognosis. The stroke work of the failing left ventricle is heavily dependent on loading conditions[50] and this may limit the value of this measurement.

It is, perhaps, unreasonable to expect too much prognostic information from measurements obtained at one point in time because this cannot allow for the rate of progression of the underlying disease. The prognosis may be affected by the aetiology of the ventricular damage. While some studies have found survival to be worse in patients with ischaemic heart disease rather than dilated cardiomyopathy[39,51], others have not have confirmed this[38].

Drug therapy

The drug treatment of chronic heart failure has been reviewed in detail elsewhere[44,52]. Diuretics remain the cornerstone of therapy. Although their value has never been studied in a clinical trial, they are obviously effective in controlling retention of fluid in patients with mild to moderate heart failure. They have been used as 'background' therapy in all the clinical trials of other agents. This should not obscure their potential for causing adverse effects, such as depletion of potassium and magnesium. Increasing the dosage of diuretics will not improve exertional symptoms of fatigue and dyspnoea once retention of fluid has been controlled[53]. Thus, excessive diuretic therapy should be avoided.

There is now reasonable evidence that treatment with digoxin is effective in heart failure when the patient remains in sinus rhythm[54]. Vasodilators and inhibitors of angiotensin-converting enzyme are now considered an essential part of the treatment of moderate to severe heart failure because of their ability to prolong survival[1,2]. The main problem with inhibitors of converting enzyme is their potential for producing hypotension and a deterioration in renal function. Although pointers to these problems, such as hyponatraemia[55], have been described, the response is unpredictable in patients with severe heart failure and treatment should be started on an in-patient basis. A variety of new oral inotropes have been investigated, but none has been established as having a role in the therapy of stable chronic heart failure[56]. Although drug therapy has the potential to prolong life in heart failure, there is also the possibility of detrimental effects. Recently it has been reported that xamoterol (a beta-blocker with partial agonist activity) increased mortality in severe heart failure[57]. Patients with left ventricular dysfunction are at risk of systemic embolism[58,59], and those who have restricted mobility are at risk of venous thrombosis and pulmonary embolism. Patients in heart failure, with no contraindication, should be anticoagulated whilst awaiting transplantation.

Arrhythmias in chronic heart failure

The importance of ventricular arrhythmias in determining the prognosis of heart failure is uncertain[38]. Sudden death is common in this population[43] but it is unclear how many of these deaths are primarily due to arrhythmias. Complex ventricular ectopy and non-sustained ventricular tachycardia are also common, but may not be predictors of death independently of ventricular dysfunction[51]. A recent study has highlighted the diverse mechanisms of sudden death in patients with advanced heart failure[60]. Sudden death is not always due to tachyarrhythmias in this population.

Patients with ventricular dysfunction are prone to adverse effects of anti-arrhythmic therapy, especially the negative inotropic effect of some drugs[61]. In addition, the anti-arrhythmic efficacy of these drugs may be reduced when a patient is in heart failure. There has been an interest, recently, in the use of amiodarone in these patients. The minimal negative inotropic effect of the drug combined with its peripheral vasodilator actions make it well tolerated from the haemodynamic point of view. Ejection fraction may improve due to a reduction in afterload[62]. A survey of amiodarone used in patients with heart failure showed that it was associated with improved survival[63]. Caution must be used, however, in interpreting the results of retrospective analyses of non-randomized treatments. This is underlined by the fact that the same study failed to show any benefit of angiotensin converting enzyme inhibitors, although a randomized clinical trial has shown a definite benefit[2]. A role for drug therapy for asymptomatic ventricular arrhythmias has not yet been established.

Patients who have experienced either an episode of symptomatic sustained ventricular tachycardia or ventricular fibrillation, not due to acute myocardial infarction, are at a high risk of sudden death. A conventional approach to these patients is to select anti-arrhythmic drugs on the basis of electrophysiological studies[64]. This is difficult to apply to patients with poor left ventricular function. An effective drug regimen may not be defined[65], and the incidence of adverse reactions is high. Although amiodarone may be effective in some patients, electrophysiological testing often fails to demonstrate the inhibition of an inducible tachycardia by this drug. This makes it difficult to predict efficacy[66].

Surgical treatment of ventricular tachycardias due to ischaemic ventricular damage has now become a realistic option[67,68]. The application of these techniques to patients with severe heart failure is limited by the increased perioperative risk with poor ventricular function. An alternative approach is the use of an automatic implantable cardioverter–defibrillator[6,69]. This has recently been found to produce encouraging results even in patients with a low ejection fraction[70]. Comparison of actual to estimated survival, based on discharge of the defibrillator, suggested a substantial prolongation of life, although there are no prospective randomized studies to confirm this finding. If a patient appears to have reasonable ventricular function when in sinus rhythm, insertion of a defibrillator, combined with conventional anti-failure therapy, may be a satisfactory approach. When malignant ventricular arrhythmias occur in the presence of very poor ventricular function, urgent transplantation is the treatment of choice.

Unstable chronic heart failure

Many patients are referred for assessment for transplantation in an unstable haemodynamic state. Intensive vasodilator therapy, guided by haemodynamic monitoring, can allow many of these patients to be established on oral therapy[71] and, if appropriate, listed for transplantation with a routine priority. When this is not possible, the patient may require intravenous inotropic or mechanical circulatory support if suitable for transplantation.

When a patient deteriorates after a period of stability, a potentially reversible factor may be found. Examples are retention of salt and water, an adverse response to vasodilators or excessive diuresis, infection, arrhythmias, or pulmonary embolism. Frequently, however, the situation is due to a further deterioration in ventricular function. If oral therapy cannot be re-established, the objective becomes to maintain the patient in a condition suitable for transplantation, preferably without resort to mechanical circulatory support. Previous assessment may help to avoid inappropriate therapy in a patient who does not want, or is unsuitable for, transplantation.

The physiology of chronic heart failure differs from that of acute heart failure. The development of ventricular dilatation helps to maintain stroke volume despite a low ejection fraction. A low arterial pressure is often well tolerated[72]. Left ventricular filling and cardiac output can often be maintained when normal filling pressures are induced by vasodilators[50]. This is because of a limited response to augmented preload in chronic heart failure, the beneficial effect of a reduced afterload and, perhaps, the reduction in mitral regurgitation associated with ventricular dilatation.

Clinical estimation of the filling pressure in the left ventricle can be very unreliable in chronic left ventricular failure[47]. The insertion of a Swan–Ganz catheter will enable precise control of therapy. The catheter should only be kept in place while it is contributing to the adjustment of therapy. This is because prolonged right heart catheterization increases the risks of infection and other catheter-related complications[73]. Intravenous diuretics and vasodilators are used as the initial lines of treatment. The objectives are to reduce left ventricular filling pressures and systemic vascular resistance while increasing the cardiac index toward normal and maintaining an adequate arterial pressure for cerebral, coronary, and renal perfusion[71].

If these goals cannot be achieved with vasodilators, inotropic drugs are required. Preservation of renal function is of paramount importance. Dopamine given at a low dosage may improve blood flow to the kidneys. The response to beta-adrenergic agonists, and analogues such as dobutamine, is often poor, probably because of down regulation of beta-receptors[74] and the development of tolerance. Recently, an inhibitor of type III phophodiesterase, enoximone[75], has been found to have some value in maintaining patients prior to transplantation without the need for mechanical support[76]. The use of vasoconstrictive inotropes (such as adrenaline and noradrenaline) is largely as a temporary measure while organizing mechanical support because of the risk of reducing organ perfusion and increasing left ventricular afterload.

Mechanical circulatory support – the 'bridge' to transplantation

If pharmacological manipulation of loading conditions and ventricular stimulation with inotropes can no longer maintain satisfactory perfusion of the vital organs, mechanical circulatory support may be considered.

The intra-aortic balloon pump has the advantages of being readily available and relatively cheap. Percutaneous insertion can be achieved in about 15 minutes to provide rapid circulatory support[77]. Although percutaneous insertion of the pump has higher incidence of vascular complications than surgical insertion, this is largely because surgical removal usually includes a routine embolectomy using a Fogarty catheter. Exploration, when indicated, after percutaneous removal of the pump achieves similar results. The incidence of infection is lower after percutaneous insertion[77]. Although intra-aortic pumps have successfully maintained patients prior to transplantation[78], the improvement that can be achieved beyond that produced by full medical therapy is often limited in this type of patient. The development of renal failure, or systemic infection, are serious complications which may preclude transplantation. The results of transplantation in such critically ill patients are inferior to those in patients without secondary organ dysfunction or infection[79].

Recently, the use of ventricular assist devices and implantable total artificial hearts to maintain patients prior to transplantation has been explored. By 1988, assist devices had been used in 74 attempts to bridge patients to transplantation. Of these patients, 54 eventually received transplants and 39 (52%) survived to be discharged from hospital[80]. An artificial heart had been used as a bridge to transplant in 111 patients. Of these, 72 had eventually received transplants with 29 survivors (26%)[81]. These results are inferior to those obtained with conventional heart transplantation[3,4]. Furthermore, the published results do not reflect the total numbers or the results of device applications. They do demonstrate, however, that bridging is technically feasible. Individual reports have indicated that good results are possible in selected patients[5,82]. In our initial experience, biventricular support has appeared to be important because it can allow a low central venous pressure to be maintained and thus enhance organ perfusion. Bleeding related to anticoagulation and increased fibrinolytic activity has proved to be a significant problem. The development of infection, thromboembolic episodes and renal failure may render the patient unsuitable for subsequent transplantation. Our current philosophy is that a patient receiving mechanical circulatory support should be maintained on support until optimal function of other organs is achieved. The criteria for accepting such a patient for transplantation should be similar to those used for assessing other candidates for transplantation.

The use of mechanical circulatory support for bridging has not been met with universal approval[83]. A fundamental objection is that, while the need for cardiac transplantations exceeds the supply of donor organs, sustaining life with such methods does not lead to a net increase either in the number of patients transplanted or lives saved. The alternative view is that patients eligible for briding will die very quickly without transplanation (or circulatory support) whereas less severely affected patients may be palliated for some time with medical therapy. Thus, bridging could increase the overall number of patient-years of life saved. The resolution of this issue depends on the results of bridging in terms of both morbidity and mortality. It is probably premature to pass judgement on these techniques because the technology is still evolving. It should be remembered that, only 10 years ago, heart transplantation was not generally accepted as a therapeutic procedure[84]. The investigational use of these techniques is contributing to the knowledge required for the development of an implantable artificial heart suitable for long-term use. The application of these methods in individual cases, however, does raise many difficult practical, ethical and financial issues.

Heart transplantation

Heart transplantation is the most effective treatment for severe ventricular failure. The 1-year survival rate at 78% is superior to the results of medical therapy (Figure 12.2). Medium-term survival is now excellent with few deaths occurring between 1 and 5 years[3,4]. Nevertheless, transplantation remains a major undertaking which generates a variety of clinical problems (Table 12.3).

The patients require life-long immunosuppression to prevent cardiac rejection. The principal drug used currently in all centres is cyclosporin[85]. This provides more effective and selective immunosuppression than the other agents available[17]. It has contributed substantially to the improvement in the results of transplantation during the last decade. Cyclosporin does have a wide variety of unwanted effects. The most serious of these is nephrotoxicity[30]. This occurs in both acute and chronic forms. The acute syndrome is reversible and dose dependent. It appears to be mediated by alterations in renal haemodynamics, and the effects can combine with other perioperative renal insults to cause acute renal failure[86]. The chronic syndrome probably also results from altered renal blood flow and ischaemia. This produces renal tubular damage and fibrosis, although renal function will improve to some extent with a reduction in dosage and levels of the drug in the blood. Fortunately, renal damage can be minimized by reducing the dose used and renal function is well preserved with regimens using lower doses[14]. There is a wide individual variation in the pharmacokinetics of cyclosporin and a number of important interactions have been recognized with various drugs. As a result, blood levels of cyclosporin must be monitored to maintain effective immunosuppression whilst minimizing toxicity[17].

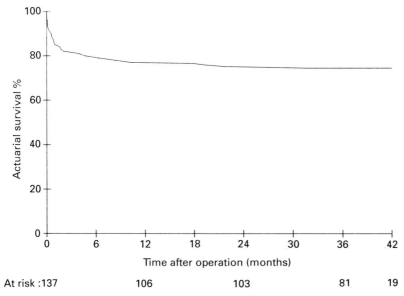

At risk :137   106   103   81   19

Figure 12.2 Actuarial survival of 137 consecutive patients undergoing heart transplantation in 1987

Cyclosporin is normally combined with other drugs for routine immunosuppression – usually corticosteroids and/or azathioprine[85]. In our unit, cyclosporin and azathioprine are used for routine immunosuppression. We attempt to minimize or avoid the use of oral steroids[11]. This avoids the side-effects of long-term treatment with steroids and may reduce the incidence of abnormalities in the metabolism of lipids and coronary arterial disease after transplantation[12,21,22]. Short courses of oral steroids are used in cases of repeated or persistent rejection, and when adequate levels of cyclosporin cannot be achieved because of renal dysfunction in the initial postoperative period[12].

Episodes of acute rejection may be suspected on clinical, electrocardiographic and echocardiographic criteria[3]. Recently there has been considerable interest in the use of Doppler echocardiographic techniques to diagnose rejection non-invasively[87]. The results of some groups have been extremely promising[88], but others have had a less satisfactory experience[89]. The 'gold standard' for the diagnosis of cardiac rejection remains the endomyocardial biopsy[90]. Acute rejection is treated with a 3-

Table 12.3 Common complications of heart transplantation

Early	Late
Acute rejection	Chronic cyclosporin nephrotoxicity
Infection – conventional and opportunistic	Hypertension
Right ventricular failure due to high pulmonary vascular resistance	Coronary arterial disease in transplanted heart
Renal failure/acute cyclosporin nephrotoxicity	Other drug toxicity and drug interactions

day course of intravenous methylprednisolone. In difficult cases this is combined with either antithymocyte globulin or the monoclonal antibody OKT3.

Bacterial infections are not a major problem with the immunosuppression regimen of cyclosporin and azathioprine. Their incidence is minimized by prophylactic administration of antibiotics, at the time of surgery[91], and they usually respond to standard antibiotic therapy. Opportunistic infections are a particular problem in the first 6 months after surgery – especially in patients who require augmented immunosuppression because of rejection[92]. The commonest serious infections are caused by cytomegalovirus and pneumocystis carinii, both of which can cause severe pneumonitis. Patients presenting with pneumonitis can usually be established by fibreoptic bronchoscopy with bronchoalveolar lavage and transbronchial biopsy. Immunocytochemical techniques[93] can be used for the rapid diagnosis of these infections. Culture of the bronchial secretions will reveal bacterial and fungal infections. Histology can give confirmation of infection with cytomegalovirus or pneumocystis and help to differentiate fungal colonization from invasive disease.

Hypertension is common after heart transplantation in patients who are treated with cyclosporin[14]. The incidence increases with time after transplantation. It is not closely linked to the dose of cyclosporin or the degree of nephrotoxicity. It had recently been demonstrated that cyclosporin increases sympathetic nervous system activity and that this effect is especially seen in heart transplant recipients, perhaps because of cardiac denervation[94]. Fortunately, most patients respond to conventional drug therapy. Beta blockers should be used with caution because of their adverse effect on the exercise response of the transplanted heart[95].

Coronary arterial disease is the most serious late complication of heart transplantation. The pathogenesis of the lesion, which differs from conventional coronary arterial disease[96], has not been established. Immune and metabolic mechanisms probably combine to damage the coronary arterial wall. The incidence of the condition appears to be influenced by the type of immunosuppression used and the level of lipids in the serum[22]. The disease may result in episodes of coronary arterial spasm, myocardial infarction, progressive ventricular dysfunction, or sudden death. Myocardial ischaemia does not usually produce chest pain in these patients because of the denervation of the transplanted heart[97]. Although the condition was originally termed 'accelerated' coronary atherosclerosis, we have observed patients with angiographic evidence of coronary arterial disease who have remained in a stable condition for several years. The prognosis of the disease is far more variable than was originally realized.

Rehabilitation after transplantation

Heart transplantation can effectively restore ventricular systolic function[98,99], but a number of other factors contribute to an abnormal physiological response to exercise (Table 12.4)[97]. Exercise capacity is below that of normal subjects[100]. The exercise response of the denervated transplanted heart is heavily dependent on circulating levels of catecholamines. The heart rate accelerates slowly and is lower than in normal subjects at peak exercise (Figures 12.3 and 12.4)[101]. Exercise training can, however, improve exercise capacity and this is associated with an increase in peak consumption of oxygen and heart rate (Figure 12.5)[102]. Some of the improvement may be due to the reversal of the effects of heart failure and deconditioning on skeletal muscle. The increased response of the heart rate suggests

Table 12.4 Factors that may influence exercise physiology after transplantation

Cardiac denervation
Deconditioning before transplantation
Effects of heart failure on skeletal muscle
Altered ventricular function:
    Donor brain death
    Preservation
    Previous rejection
    Cyclosporin associated fibrosis
Hypertension
Drug therapy

For references see reference[97].

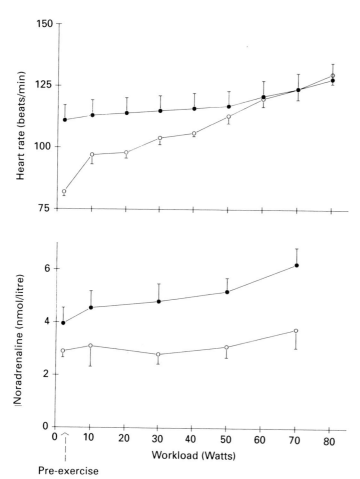

Figure 12.3 Heart rate (top) and noradrenaline levels (bottom) during progressive dynamic exercise on a cycle ergometer. Heart transplant recipients (●———●) compared with matched normal controls (○———○). Noradrenaline levels are higher in the transplant group suggesting an increased level of sympathetic activity. Circulating catecholamines mediate the heart rate response during exercise in the transplanted, denervated, heart which is supersensitive to endogenous catecholamines. Initial heart rates are higher in the transplant group due to the lack of vagal tone and the influence of circulating catecholamines[97] (Reproduced from reference[101], by permission.)

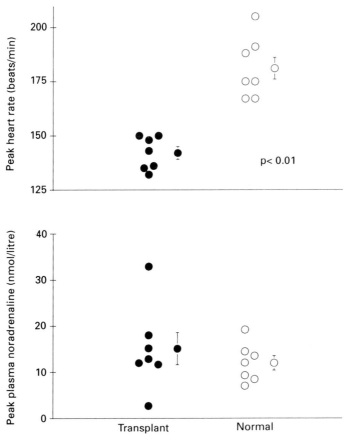

Figure 12.4 Peak heart rate (top) and noradrenaline levels (bottom) at the end of symptom limited dynamic exercise. The maximum workload achieved by the transplant recipients (●——●) was less than that of the normal controls (○——○) at 102 ± 8 versus 170 ± 10 W, respectively. Despite a similar level of noradrenaline, and hence sympathetic activity, in the two groups the heart transplant recipients reach lower peak heart rates due to cardiac denervation (Reproduced from reference [101], by permission.)

that central haemodynamic changes may also be important. Although the mechanisms underlying the response of the denervated heart to exercise training have not been fully evaluated, a programme of exercise training clearly can contribute to a physical rehabilitation after heart transplantation. The great majority of patients achieve a good level of rehabilitation and quality of life after heart transplantation.

Conclusions

While important advances have been made in the medical management of heart failure, the mortality remains high in patients with severe ventricular dysfunction. Cardiac transplantation has become established as a highly effective treatment for end-stage myocardial failure. Transplantation is a complex procedure which has

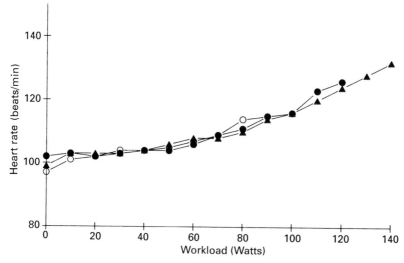

Figure 12.5 Example of the exercise training response of an orthotopic heart transplant recipient participating in a cardiac rehabilitation programme. There was a progressive increase in the peak workload achieved in tests performed at 3 (O——O), 6 (●——●) and 12 (▲——▲) months (90, 120 and 140 W, respectively). This was associated with an increase in the heart rate at peak exercise but no evidence of a training bradycardia at sub-maximal workloads

generated a new set of challenges for the cardiologist and cardiac surgeon. The limited supply of donor organs complicates the management of the candidate for heart transplantation. The unpredictable nature of severe heart failure makes it difficult to assign priorities to candidates and patients continue to die whilst awaiting transplantation. This has led to the application of systems for mechanical circulatory support to maintain deteriorating patients until a transplant can be performed. This aspect of transplantation must still be regarded as investigational, and raises a variety of practical and ethical problems.

Transplantation will only be able to meet the needs of a small proportion of patients with heart failure because of the limited supply of donor organs. Further improvements in drug therapy may be achieved but other approaches are needed. The next few years will probably see an increasing interest in the use of skeletal muscle for circulatory support[103,104] and further progress towards a totally implantable artificial heart for long-term use and towards cardiac xenotransplantation.

References

1. Cohn, J.N., Archibald, D.G., Ziesche, S., *et al.* Effect of vasodilator therapy on mortality in chronic congestive heart failure. Results of a Veterans Administration Cooperative Study. *N. Engl. J. Med.*, **314**, 1547–1552, 1986
2. The CONSENSUS trial study group. Effects of enalapril on mortality in severe congestive heart failure. *N. Engl. J. Med.*, **316**, 1429–1435, 1987
3. Banner, N.R., Khaghani, A., Fitzgerald, M., *et al.* The expanding role of cardiac transplantation. In *Assisted Circulation 3* (ed. F. Unger), Springer Verlag, Berlin, pp. 448–467, 1989
4. Kriett J.M. and Kaye, M.P. The registry of the international society for heart transplantation: seventh official report 1990. *J. Heart Transplant.*, **9**, 323–330, 1990

5. Farrar, D.J., Hill, J.D., Gray, L.A., *et al.* Heterotopic prosthetic ventricles as a bridge to cardiac transplantation. A multicentre study in 29 patients. *N. Engl. J. Med.*, **318**, 333–340, 1988
6. Mirowski, M. The automatic implantable cardioverter defibrillator: an overview. *J. Am. Coll. Cardiol.*, **6**, 461–466, 1985
7. Evans, R.W., Mannihen, D.L., Garrison, L.P., *et al.* Donor availability as the primary determinant of the future of heart transplantation. *J. Am. Med. Assoc.*, **225**, 1892–1898, 1986
8. Popp, R.L. Echocardiography. *N. Engl. J. Med.*, **323**, 101–109, 165–172, 1990
9. Douglas, P.S., Morrow, R. Ioll, A. and Reichek, N. Left ventricular shape, afterload and survival in idiopathic dilated cardiomyopathy. *J. Am. Coll. Cardiol.*, **13**, 311–315, 1989
10. Aravot, D.J., Banner, N.R., Madden, B., *et al.* Primary cardiac tumours – is there a place for cardiac transplantation? *Eur. J. Cardiothorac. Surg.*, **3**, 521–524, 1989
11. Yacoub, M.H., Alivizatos, P.A., Khaghani, A. and Mitchell, A. The use of cyclosporin azathioprine and antithymocyte globulin with or without low dose steroids for immunosuppression of cardiac transplant patients. *Transplant Proc.*, **17**, 221–222, 1985
12. Banner, N.R., Fitzgerald, M., Khaghani, A., *et al.* Cardiac transplantation at Harefield Hospital. In *Clinical Transplants* (ed. E.I. Terasaki), UCLA Tissue Typing Laboratory, Los Angeles, pp. 17–26, 1987
13. Hastillo, A. and Hess, M.L. Selection of patients for cardiac transplantation. In *Cardiac Transplantation* (ed. E. Thompson), F.A. Davis, Philadelphia, pp. 107–120, 1990
14. Ozdogan, E., Banner, N., Fitzgerald, M., *et al.* Factors influencing the development of hypertension following cardiac transplantation. *J. Heart Transpalnt.* (in press), 1990
15. Young, J.N., Yazbeck, J., Esposito, G., *et al.* The influence of acute preoperative pulmonary infarction on the results of heart transplantation. *J. Heart Transplant.*, **5**, 20–22, 1986
16. McAleer-Rhenman, M.J., Rhenman, B., Icenogle, T.B., *et al.* Diabetes mellitus in heart transplantation. *J. Heart Transplant.*, **7**, 64, 1988
17. Kahan, B.D. Cyclosporin. *N. Engl. J. Med.*, **321**, 1725–1738, 1989
18. Aravot, D., Banner, N., Khaghani, A., *et al.* Cardiac transplantation in patients with present or past malignant neoplasms (abstract). *Br. Heart J.*, **61**, 464, 1989
19. Aravot, D.J., Banner, N.R., Khaghani, A., *et al.* Cardiac transplantation in the seventh decade of life. *Am. J. Cardiol.*, **63**, 90–93, 1989
20. Yacoub, M.H., Mankad, P. and Ledingham, S. Donor procurement and surgical techniques for cardiac transplantation. *Semin. Thoracic Cardiovasc. Surg.*, **2**, 153–161, 1990
21. Barbir, M., Banner, N.R., Trayner, I., *et al.* High prevalence of lipid and lipoprotein abnormalities in heart transplant recipients (abstract). *Eur. Heart J.*, **10 Abstract Suppl.** 32, 1989
22. Barbir, M., Banner, N., Reid, C.J., *et al.* Influence of lipid abnormalities on the development of coronary artery disease after cardiac transplantation (abstract). *Br. Heart J.*, **61**, 462, 1989
23. Bolli, R. Mechanisms of myocardial 'stunning'. *Circulation*, **82**, 723–738, 1990
24. Dilsizian, V., Rocco, T.P., Freedman, N.M.T., *et al.* Enhanced detection of ischaemic but viable myocardium by the reinjection of thallium after stress redistribution imaging. *N. Engl. J. Med.*, **323**, 141–146, 1990
25. Tillisch, J., Brunken, R., Marshall, R., *et al.* Reversibility of cardiac wall motion abnormalities predicted by positron tomography. *N. Engl. J. Med.*, **314**, 884–888, 1986
26. Conner, R., Hosenpud, J.D., Norman, D.J., *et al.* Heart transplantation for cardiac amyloidosis: successful 1 year outcome despite recurrence of the disease. *J. Heart Transplant.*, **7**, 165, 1988
27. Stolf, N.A.G., Higushi, L., Bocchi, E., *et al.* Heart transplantation in patients with Chagas' cardiomyopathy. *J. Heart Transplant.*, **6**, 307–312, 1987
28. Kong, G., Madden, B., Spyrou, S., *et al.* Response of recurrent giant cell myocarditis in a transplanted heart to intensive immunosuppression. *Eur. Heart J.* (in press), 1990
29. Yacoub, M.H., Banner, N.R., Khaghani, A., Fitzgerald, M., Madden, B., Tsang, V., Radley-Smith, R., Hodson, M. Heart–lung transplantation for Cystic Fibrosis and subsequent domino heart transplantation. *J. Heart Transplant.* (in press), 1990
30. Neild, G.H. Cyclosporin nephrotoxicity. *Semin. Thoracic Cardiovasc. Surg.*, **2**, 198–203, 1990
31. McClosky, D., Festenstein, H., Banner, N., *et al.* The effect of HLA lymphocytotoxic antibody status and cross match result on cardiac transplant survival. *Transplant Proc.*, **21**, 2548–2550, 1989
32. Khaghani, A., Yacoub, M., McCloskey, D., *et al.* The influence of HLA matching, donor/recipient sex and incidence of acute rejection on survival in cardiac allograft recipients receiving cyclosporin and azathioprine. *Transplant Proc.*, **21**, 799–800, 1989
33. Mackinson, S., Burnett, A.K., Crawford, R.J., *et al.* Seronegative blood products prevent primary cytomegalovirus infection after bone marrow transplantation. *J. Clin. Pathol.*, **41**, 948–950, 1988

34. Stevenson, L.W., Fowler, M.B., Schroeder, J.S., et al. Poor survival in patients with idiopathic cardiomyopathy considered too well for transplantation. Am. J. Med., **83**, 871–876, 1987

35. Cohn, J.N. and Rector, T.S. Prognosis of congestive heart failure and predictors of mortality. Am. J. Cardiol., **62 Suppl. A**, 25A–30A, 1988

36. Diaz, R.A., Obasohan, A. and Oakley, C.M. Prediction of outcome in dilated cardiomyopathy. Br. Heart J., **58**, 393–399, 1987

37. Unverferth, D.V., Magorien, R.D., Moeschberger, M.L., et al. Factors influencing 1 year mortality in dilated cardiomyopathy. Am. J. Cardiol., **54**, 147–152, 1984

38. Wilson, J.R., Schwartz, S., Sutton, M. St. J., et al. Prognosis in severe heart failure: relation to haemodynamic measurements and ventricular ectopic activity. J. Am. Coll. Cardiol., **2**, 403–410, 1983

39. Franciosa, J.A., Wilen, M., Ziesche, S. and Cohn, J. Survival in men with chronic left ventricular failure due to either coronary artery disease or idiopathic dilated cardiomyopathy. Am. J. Cardiol., **51**, 831–836, 1983

40. Olshausen, K.V., Stienen, U., Math, D., et al. Long term prognostic significance of ventricular arrhythmias in idiopathic dilated cardiomyopathy. Am. J. Cardiol., **61**, 146–151, 1988

41. Slinker, B.K. and Glantz, S.A. Multiple regression for physiological data analysis: the problem of multicollinearity. Am. J. Physiol., **249**, R1–R12, 1985

42. Moss, A.J. and Benhorin, J. Prognosis and management after first myocardial infarction. N. Engl. J. Med., **322**, 743–753, 1990

43. Packer, P. Sudden unexplained death in patients with congestive heart failure: a second frontier. Circulation, **72**, 681–685, 1985

44. Cohn, J.N. Current therapy of the failing hearts. Circulation, **78**, 1099–1107, 1988

45. Gordon, E.P., Schnittger, I., Fitzgerald, P.J., et al. Reproducibility of left ventricular volumes by two-dimensional echocardiography. J. Am. Coll. Cardiol., **2**, 506–513, 1983

46. Stevenson, W.G., Stevenson, L.W., Weiss, J. and Tillisch, J.H. Inducible ventricular arrhythmias and sudden death during vasodilator therapy of severe heart failure. Am. Heart J., **116**, 1147–1454, 1988

47. Stevenson, L.W. and Perloff, J. The limited reliability of physical signs in estimating haemodynamics in chronic heart failure. J. Am. Med. Assoc., **261**, 884–888, 1989

48. Packer, M., Lee, W.H., Medina, N., et al. Prognostic importance of immediate haemodynamic response to nifedipine in patients with severe left ventricular dysfunction. J. Am. Coll. Cardiol., **10**, 1303–1311, 1987

49. Tan, L.B. Cardiac pumping capability and prognosis in heart failure. Lancet, **ii**, 1360–1363, 1986

50. Stevenson, L.W. and Tillisch, J.H. Maintenance of cardiac output with normal filling pressures in patients with dilated heart failure. Circulation, **74**, 1303–1308, 1986

51. Likoff, M.J., Chandler, S.L. and Kay, H.R. Clinical determinants of mortality in congestive heart failure secondary to idiopathic dilated or ischaemic cardiomyopathy. Am. J. Cardiol., **59**, 634–638, 1987

52. Packer, M. Vasodilator and inotropic drugs for the treatment of chronic heart failure: distinguishing hype from hope. J. Am. Coll. Cardiol., **12**, 1299–1317, 1988

53. Poole-Wilson, P.A. and Buller, N.P. Causes of symptoms in chronic congestive heart failure and implications for treatment. Am. J. Cardiol., **62**, 31A–34A, 1988

54. Smith, T.W. Digitalis – mechanisms of action and clinical use. N. Engl. J. Med., **318**, 358–365, 1988

55. Packer, M., Lee, W.H., Kessler, P.D., et al. Identification of hyponataemia as a risk factor for the development of functional renal insufficiency during converting enzyme inhibition in severe chronic heart failure. J. Am. Coll. Cardiol., **10**, 837–844, 1987

56. Colucci, W.S., Wright, R.F. and Braunwald, E. New positive inotropic agents in the treatment of congestive heart failure. Mechanisms of action and recent clinical developments. N. Engl. J. Med., **314**, 290–299, 349–358, 1986

57. The xamoterol in severe heart failure study group. Xamoterol in severe heart failure. Lancet, **336**, 1–6, 1990

58. Fuster, V., Gersh, B.J., Giulini, E.R., et al., The natural history of idiopathic dilated cardiomyopathy. Am. J. Cardiol., **47**, 525–531, 1981

59. Stratton, J.R. and Resnick, A.D. Increased embolic risk in patients with left ventricular thrombi. Circulation, **75**, 1004–1011, 1987

60. Luu, M., Stevenson, W.G., Stevenson, L.W., et al. Diverse mechanisms of unexpected cardiac arrest in advanced heart failure population. Circulation, **80**, 1675–1680, 1989

61. Wilson, J.R. Use of antiarrhythmic drugs in patients with heart failure: clinical efficacy, haemodynamic results and relation to survival. Circulation, **75 Suppl. IV**, 64–73, 1987

62. Hamer, A.W.F., Arkles, L.B. and Johns, J.A. Beneficial effects of low dose amiodarone in patients with congestive heart failure: a placebo controlled trial. *J. Am. Coll. Cardiol.*, **14**, 1768–1774, 1989

63. Cleland, J.G., Dargie, H.J. and Ford, I. Mortality in heart failure: clinical variables of prognostic value. *Br. Heart J.*, **58**, 572–582, 1987

64. Swerdlow, C.D., Winkle, R.A. and Mason, J.W. Determinants of survival in patients with ventricular tachyarrhythmias. *N. Engl. J. Med.*, **308**, 1436–1442, 1983

65. Poll, D.S., Marchlinski, F.E., Buxton, A.E., *et al.* Sustained ventricular tachycardia in patients with idiopathic dilated cardiomyopathy: electrophysiologic testing and lack of response to antiarrhythmic therapy. *Circulation*, **70**, 451–456, 1984

66. Yazaki, Y., Haffajee, C.I., Gold, R.L., *et al.* Electrophysiological predictors of long term outcome with amiodarone for refractory ventricular tachycardia secondary to coronary artery disease. *Am. J. Cardiol.*, **60**, 293–297, 1987

67. Cox, J.L. Ventricular tachycardia surgery: a review of the first decade and a suggested contemporary approach. *Semin. Thoracic Cardiovasc. Surg.*, **1**, 97–103, 1989

68. Hargrove, W.C. Surgery for ischaemic ventricular tachycardia – operative techniques and long-term results. *Semin. Thoracic Cardiovasc. Surg.*, **1**, 83–87, 1989

69. Hammon, J.W. The role of the automatic implantable cardioverter-defibrillator in the treatment of ventricular tachycardia. *Semin. Thoracic Cardiovasc. Surg.*, **1**, 88–96, 1989

70. Tchou, P.J., Kadri, N., Anderson, J., *et al.* Automatic implantable cardioverter defibrillators and survival in left ventricular dysfunction and malignant ventricular arrhythmias. *Ann. Intern. Med.*, **109**, 529–534, 1988

71. Stevenson, L.W., Dracup, K.A. and Tillisch, J.H. Efficacy of medical therapy tailored for severe congestive heart failure in patients transferred for urgent cardiac transplantation. *Am. J. Cardiol.*, **63**, 461–464, 1989

72. Weber, K.T., Janicki, J.S., Campbell, C. and Replogle, R. Pathophysiology of acute and chronic cardiac failure. *Am. J. Cardiol.*, **60 Suppl. C**, 3C–9C, 1987

73. Robin, E.D. The cult of the Swan Ganz catheter. *Ann. Intern. Med.*, **103**, 445–449, 1985

74. Bristow, M.R., Ginsburg, R., Minobe, W., *et al.* Decreased catecholamine sensitivity and beta-adrenergic-receptor density in failing human hearts. *N. Engl. J. Med.*, **307**, 205–211, 1982

75. Dage, R.C., Kariya, T., Hsieh, C.P., *et al.* Pharmacology of enoximone. *Am. J. Cardiol.*, **60**, 10C–14C, 1987

76. Loisance, D., Dubois Rande, J.L., Tarral, Ph.D.A. Enoximone therapy: an alternative strategy to temporary mechanical support. In *Assisted Circulation 3* (ed. F. Unger), Springer Verlag, Berlin, pp. 304–312, 1989

77. Goldberg, M.J., Rubenfire, M., Kantowitz, A., *et al.* Intraaortic balloon pump insertion: a randomised study comparing percutaneous and surgical techniques. *J. Am. Coll. Cardiol.*, **9**, 515–523, 1987

78. O'Connell, J.B., Renlund, D.G., Robinson, J.A., *et al.* Effect of preoperative haemodynamic support on survival after cardiac transplantation. *Circulation*, **78 Suppl. III**, 78–82, 1988

79. Mulchahy, D., Wright, C., Mockus, L., *et al.* Cardiac transplantation in severely ill patients requiring intensive support in hospital. *Br. Med. J. (Clin. Res.)*, **296**, 817–819, 1988

80. Unger, F. Ventricular assist devices: possibilities and limits. In *Assisted Circulation 3* (ed. F. Unger), Springer Verlag, Berlin, pp. 97–102, 1989

81. Unger, F. The use of artificial hearts for bridging to transplantation. In *Assisted Circulation 3* (ed. F. Unger), Springer Verlag, Berlin, pp. 245–246, 1989

82. Griffith, B.P., Hardesty, R.L., Kormos, R.L., *et al.* Temporary use of the Jarvick-7 total artificial heart before transplantation. *N. Engl. J. Med.*, **316**, 130–134, 1987

83. Annas, G.J. Temporary use of the artificial heart before transplantation (letter). *N. Engl. J. Med.*, **317**, 314–315, 1987

84. Leaf, A. The MGH trustees say no to heart transplants. *N. Engl. J. Med.*, **302**, 1087–1088, 1980

85. Renlund, D.G., O'Connell, J.B. and Bristow, M.R. Strategies of immunosuppression in cardiac transplantation. *Semin. Thoracic Cardiovasc. Surg.*, **2**, 181–188, 1990

86. Goldman, M.H., Barnhart, G., Mohanakumar, T., *et al.* Cyclosporine in cardiac transplantation. *Surg. Clin. N. Am.*, **65**, 637–659, 1985

87. Valantine, H.A., Fowler, M.B., Hunt, S.A., *et al.* Changes in Doppler echocardiographic indices of left ventricular function as potential markers of acute rejection. *Circulation*, **76 Suppl. V**, V86–V92, 1987

88. Desruennes, M., Corcos, T., Cabrol, A., *et al.* Doppler echocardiography for the diagnosis of acute cardiac allograft rejection. *J. Am. Coll. Cardiol.*, **12**, 63–70, 1988

89. Forster, T., McGhie, J., Rijsterborgh, H., *et al.* Can we assess the changes of ventricular filling resulting from acute allograft rejection with Doppler echocardiography? *J. Heart Transplant.*, **7**, 430–434, 1988

90. Billingham, M.E. Diagnosis of cardiac rejection by endomyocardial biopsy. *J. Heart Transplant.*, **1**, 25–30, 1982
91. Khaghani, A., Martin, M., Fitzgerald, M., *et al.* Cefotaxime and flucloxacillin as antibiotic prophylaxis in cardiac transplantation. *Drugs*, **35 Suppl. 2**, 124–126, 1988
92. Dummer, J.S. Infectious complications of transplantation. In *Cardiac Transplantation* (ed. M.E. Thompson), F.A. Davis, Philadelphia, pp. 163–178, 1990
93. Griffith, P.D., Panjwani, D.D., Stirk, P.R., *et al.* Rapid diagnosis of cytomegalovirus infection in immunocompromised patients by detection of early antigen fluorescent foci. *Lancet*, **ii**, 1242–1245, 1987
94. Scherrer, U., Vissing, S.F., Morgan, B.J., *et al.* Cyclosporin induced sympathetic activation and hypertension after heart transplantation. *N. Engl. J. Med.*, **323**, 693–699, 1990
95. Bexton, R.S., Milne, J.R., Cory-Pearce, R., *et al.* Effect of Beta-blockade on exercise response after cardiac transplantation. *Br. Heart J.*, **49**, 584–588, 1983
96. Gao, S-Z, Hunt, S.A. and Schroeder, J.S. Accelerated transplant coronary artery disease. *Semin. Thoracic Cardiovasc. Surg.* (in press), 1991
97. Banner, N.R. and Yacoub, M.H. Physiology of the orthotopic cardiac transplant recipient. *Semin. Thoracic Cardiovasc. Surg.* (in press), 1990
98. Borow, K.M., Neumann, A., Arensman, F.W. and Yacoub, M.H. Left ventricular contractility and contractile reserve in humans after cardiac transplantation. *Circulation*, **71**, 866–872, 1985
99. Reid, C.J. and Yacoub, M.H. Determinants of left ventricular function 1 year after cardiac transplantation. *Br. Heart J.*, **59**, 397–402, 1988
100. Banner, N.R., Lloyd, M.H., Hamilton, R.D., *et al.* Cardiopulmonary response to dynamic exercise after heart and combined heart lung transplantation. *Br. Heart J.*, **61**, 215–223, 1989
101. Banner, N.R., Patel, N., Cox, A.P., *et al.* Altered sympathoadrenal response to dynamic exercise in cardiac transplant recipients. *Cardiovasc. Res.*, **23**, 965–972, 1989
102. Kavanagh, T., Yacoub, M.H., Mertens, D.J., *et al.* Cardiorespiratory responses to exercise training after othotopic cardiac transplantation. *Circulation*, **77**, 162–171, 1988
103. Hagege, A., Desnos, M., Chachques, J.C., *et al.* Preliminary report: follow up after dynamic cardiomyopasty. *Lancet*, **335**, 1122–1124, 1990
104. Pattison, C.W., Cumming, D.V.E., Williamson, A., *et al.* Aortic counterpulsation for up to 28 days using autologous latissimus dorsi in sheep. *J. Thorac. Cardiovasc. Surg.* (in press), 1991

13

Electrophysiological basis of sudden cardiac death

Edward Rowland

Introduction

Sudden unexpected death has been described as of epidemic proportions. In the USA, sudden death claims between 200 000 and 400 000 victims per year of the 700 000 annual deaths resulting from coronary arterial disease. The number afflicted in the UK is between 50 000 and 100 000. The prevalence of coronary arterial disease makes sudden unexpected death the most common cause of death.

It has been established that most victims of sudden cardiac death are in ventricular fibrillation rather than electrical asystole at the time of arrest, while numerous paramedic and/or community programmes have shown the value of cardiopulmonary resuscitation when instituted by bystanders, and the importance of the availability of defibrillation for rescuing these victims[1–6]. Experience pioneered in Belfast and subsequently developed in several centres in the USA, notably Seattle and Miami, demonstrated the value of early defibrillation and the potential for significant numbers to be 'rescued' and returned to active lives[3,5,7,8]. Further developments, and refinements of these community programmes, have demonstrated the increased rates of salvage achievable by enhanced programmes designed to respond more quickly and able to deliver with a shorter delay corrective therapy by trained or community personnel.

Complementary and corroborative information concerning the events immediately preceding and at the time of cardiac arrest has clarified some aspects of the mechanism of sudden cardiac death, but have left many questions unanswered. Associated in most instances with coronary arterial disease, the majority of victims do not have acute myocardial infarction. Although recent series have attested to an improved outcome for survivors of cardiac arrest, certain subgroups, particularly those with sudden cardiac death unrelated to myocardial infarction have a high rate of recurrent events[3,9]. It has also become clear that the degree of left ventricular impairment, and the presence of inducible ventricular arrhythmias in the survivors, are independent predictors for further events[10].

Epidemiological studies have provided information on the characteristics of patients dying suddenly as well as clarifying the risk factors. Post-mortem studies have revealed the cardiac abnormalities that provide the setting for sudden cardiac death as well as defining the extent, severity and pathological processes leading to cardiac arrest in those with coronary arterial disease. But it has been studies of the electrocardiogram at the time of arrest, and electrophysiological investigation of those surviving cardiac arrest, that has provided the insights into the relationship between the underlying or associated heart disease and the occurrence of electrical instability that appears to occur in most episodes of sudden cardiac death. Furthermore, while sudden cardiac death occurs, in most cases, in the context of coronary arterial disease, it is a frequent consequence of other forms of heart disease. Whether the same electrophysiological features are shared in common, or whether the implications for antiarrhythmic management are similarly relevant, has not been fully clarified.

Definition

A precise definition of sudden death has not been universally agreed. In general, it is taken either to encompass death that occurs instantaneously, or else death that occurs up to 24 hours after the onset of symptoms. The 1979 Task Force of the International Society and Federation of Cardiology and World Health Organisation on Nomenclature and Criteria for diagnosis of Ischaemic Heart Disease opted to define cardiac arrest, and thereby allow 'sudden death' to be applied where either resuscitation failed or was not attempted[11]. This definition had the justification of taking cardiac arrest, which is a more precise clinical manifestation, as its basis and implying that the interval between time of death and onset of symptoms should be recorded. It is debatable whether an interval as long as 24 hours remains tenable for the diagnosis of sudden death. The diagnosis seems tenable, none the less, when death, as a natural process, occurs unexpectedly and develops rapidly. An equally compelling area for precise definition concerns the survivors of sudden cardiac death – given the rapidly expanding use of cardiopulmonary resuscitation in the community and the increasing number of studies performed on survivors of sudden cardiac death. The majority of studies have included as a prerequisite only those who have required direct current countershock for ventricular fibrillation or sustained hypotensive ventricular tachycardia. The necessity for a precise definition in order to classify death in response to antiarrhythmic medication has led to a more rigorous definition that attempts to define death as being likely to be arrhythmic or nonarrhythmic based on whether it was witnessed, whether there were associated symptoms and the time from the onset of symptoms to death[12]. These guidelines, developed into a classification, were promulgated by the Cardiac Arrhythmia Pilot Study Investigators and subsequently used for the Cardiac Arrhythmia Suppression Trial[13].

Pathological studies

Observations from epidemiological and pathological studies indicate that sudden cardiac death is most frequently due to coronary arterial disease, the majority of cases showing severe occlusive disease of major coronary arteries[14–16]. Recent occlusive vascular lesions are uncommon. Indeed, only 10–30% have histological evidence of associated acute myocardial infarction. Of the remaining cases, 40% have mural thrombi alone, while 25% have no evident thrombus. The presence of thrombus appears to correlate with single vessel disease, acute infarction and prodromal symptoms, while absence of thrombus is associated with extensive coronary arterial lesions, previous evidence of ischaemic heart disease, and the presence of old infarction. Corroborative evidence for these pathological observations has been derived from the study of survivors of sudden cardiac deaths. These studies have not only demonstrated the common findings of significant coronary arterial disease, despite the absence of prior suggestive history, but also confirmed the low incidence of associated acute myocardial infarction[17,18].

From the clinical standpoint, the relationship between sudden cardiac death and coronary arterial disease exhibits two distinct patterns, of differing prognostic and clinical implications, based on the presence or absence of associated myocardial infarction. It is, however, not always possible to separate patients resuscitated from sudden death clearly into these two groups, since a minority will not demonstrate clearly whether infarction preceded death or arose as a consequence of arrhythmia.

Far fewer victims of sudden cardiac death reveal other forms of underlying heart disease although significant numbers have dilated or hypertrophic cardiomyopathy or aortic valvar disease. Rarer causes are those with right ventricular dysplasia, long QT syndrome, other various congenital cardiac malformations, and the Wolff–Parkinson–White syndrome. The last diagnosis would have to have been known prior to death, as it would only be discovered post-mortem as a consequence of detailed dissection and histological examination of the entire atrioventricular junction. In very rare circumstances, a so-called electrical cardiomyopathy character-ized by repetitive ventricular arrhythmias without ventricular dysfunction may be the cause. While such pathological associations are well known, the relationship between the pathological state and physiological behaviour, particularly electrophy-siological, is poorly understood.

Sudden cardiac death in ischaemic heart disease

Ischaemic heart disease represents one of the major scourges of the Western world, being not only the leading cause of sudden death but also, because of its various forms of expression, being a major cause of morbidity. While the predominant expression may be angina, persistent or transient electrical abnormalities play an important role in all aspects of the disease. As the epidemic of coronary arterial disease has been growing, our knowledge of the electrical consequences of the problem has been expanding dramatically. This has developed particularly from the ability to monitor the electrocardiogram during and following the development of chest pain, as well as for prolonged periods in the chronic phase of ischaemic heart disease.

Following directly from these observations has been the realization that many patients 'rescued' from the potentially fatal consequences of their ischaemic disease may have had electrical complications that may well be amenable to therapeutic interventions. While such capabilities have clearly been demonstrated in the context of acute myocardial infarction, there remain many other important areas in which the benefits of therapeutic intervention have not been proven.

The electrical consequences of coronary arterial disease are dominated by the vast problem of sudden cardiac death. Approximately 60% of the annual deaths from coronary arterial disease occur suddenly. Whether viewed from the community (sudden cardiac death accounts for approximately 20% of all natural fatalities) or from the hospital coronary unit (60% of all those dying suddenly following myocardial infarction do so in the first hour), the problem is of immense proportions.

Sudden death in association with acute myocardial infarction

The symptoms preceding sudden death are apparently identical with those who have acute coronary occlusion without fatal consequences. The prodromal symptoms result in many of these patients seeking medical attention and, thus, being admitted to hospital. There remain, however, a majority of those with warning symptoms who either do not seek medical advice or who die before they are admitted to hospital. It has been demonstrated that 40% of cases of sudden death occur within 4 h of the onset of chest pain[19]. Thereafter, the incidence of sudden death falls abruptly, illustrating that a substantial delay in patients reaching hospital will result in the major proportion of lethal consequences occurring out of hospital, rather than in the coronary care units which are designed specifically to deal with them.

The modes of sudden cardiac death in the context of acute myocardial infarction may be ventricular fibrillation, bradycardia or electromechanical dissociation. Primary ventricular fibrillation (that is, fibrillation occurring in the absence of cardiac failure) tends to occur in younger patients, particularly when there is a relatively large area of anterior damage. Paradoxically, these patients seem to retain good cardiac function. Their prognosis after resuscitation, which is generally straightforward, is similar to those with uncomplicated infarction. Recurrences are unlikely and are limited to the ensuing 2–3 days.

Asystole or complete heart block are the primary mode of cardiac arrest in relatively few patients with acute myocardial infarction. A similar temporal pattern occurs with these arrhythmias, as is seen with primary ventricular tachycardia – the majority of cases occurring within a short time of the onset of symptoms. Those with inferior infarction, however, develop bradyarrhythmias more commonly than those with infarction at other sites.

The least common form of sudden death, and the least amenable to treatment, is electromechanical dissociation. It may occur as a primary event or may follow resuscitation from secondary ventricular fibrillation complicating severe cardiac failure. Although satisfactory ventricular depolarizations are present at first, there is no associated cardiac output and, eventually, even cardiac electrical activity ceases.

Further subgroups of patients at risk of sudden death are those with severe cardiac failure or shock (secondary ventricular fibrillation) and a minority of those in the convalescent phase of acute myocardial failure. The outlook for those with secondary fibrillation is dismal. Even if resuscitation is successful, advancing cardiac failure usually exerts its toll within weeks. Sudden death occurs during convalescence in an appreciable number – up to 20% of those dying in hospital may succumb in this phase[20]. As the initial course of their stay in hospital has usually been uncomplicated, these patients have often been transferred to general wards. Ventricular fibrillation is the almost universal mode of death in these patients, who do have certain features that are associated with this risk. Amongst these are anteroseptal infarction (especially when accompanied by right bundle branch block), development of new bundle branch block, complex ventricular arrhythmia (soon but not immediately after infarction) and persisting sinus tachycardia. Approaches to the appropriate treatment of these patients have floundered on the inability of antiarrhythmic drugs to prevent the arrhythmia. At the present time, close monitoring and observation of those considered to be at greatest risk offer the only useful approach.

While resuscitation is effective in the vast majority, a preferred approach would be primary prevention. But there is an immediate problem – should all patients receive prophylaxis or can we identify the minority at high risk? The concept of warning arrhythmias has been developed in the expectation that ventricular fibrillation will be preceded by a period of increasing arrhythmogenicity. None of the arrhythmias postulated, however, has been shown to have sufficient sensitivity or specificity. Complex ventricular extrasystoles do indeed occur with increasing frequency prior to the onset of fibrillation, but they occur in equal frequency in those not prone to this lethal consequence. They have no value, therefore, as warning signs[21]. Also, a significant proportion of those who do go on to develop fibrillation do not have preceding arrhythmias. The only possible exception is an increase in the frequency of R on T ventricular extrasystoles within the 12 h preceding the onset of ventricular fibrillation, although sophisticated electronic monitoring of the electrocardiogram is required to show a slowly developing trend that the eye can easily miss[22].

So if there is no satisfactory warning sign that ventricular fibrillation is about to occur, can prophylactic antiarrhythmic therapy prevent it? Lignocaine has led the way, and has been shown to reduce the incidence of primary ventricular fibrillation (although mortality was the same in the control group) when used in the coronary care unit[23]. Other studies have failed to demonstrate a significant reduction in mortality although, in most studies, the overall trend has been towards a reduction[24,25].

When used as mass prophylaxis (being administered to all admissions to the coronary care unit in order to protect a small minority) there clearly has to be considerable concern about toxicity. Additionally, patients may be admitted to coronary care units with suspected infarction and prove not to have had an infarction but will have still received lignocaine. Both cardiac and neuronal toxicity are significant problems with lignocaine. None of the newer antiarrhythmic drugs has demonstrated a significant reduction in the incidence of ventricular fibrillation.

Prophylactic antiarrhythmic drugs given in the coronary care unit suffer the same drawback as monitoring itself – if there is significant delay between onset of pain and hospital admission, the majority of salvable cases have already been missed. Interest has developed, therefore, in the administration of these drugs soon after the onset of chest pain by community paramedics[26]. Provided that increased recruitment of those at-risk is not accompanied by an increased in the number who subsequently prove not to have had an infarction, this approach seems highly desirable.

Sudden death remote from myocardial infarction

Although the risk of sudden death declines within the increasing duration after infarction, mortality during the first year is in the region of 10%. Two directions have been followed in an attempt to deal with the problem. Perhaps the most impressive has been the development of community-based programmes for resuscitation aimed at getting experienced medical and paramedical staff to a victim of sudden death within the vital seconds of an event[15]. Such an approach has the benefit of incorporating the community in general more closely into health care, but has the major limitation of dealing with the problem after the event. The second approach, that of identifying those at risk of sudden death and using prophylactic measures to prevent the lethal outcome, is clearly preferable. Various markers have been evaluated for such a role.

Ambulatory monitoring has revealed that many patients who have had myocardial infarction have ventricular arrhythmia that occurs spontaneously during normal daily activities[27]. The most frequently observed arrhythmia is the presence of ventricular extrasystoles, the incidence depending on the duration of monitoring. In all the studies that have examined this relationship, there is an increased prevalence of sudden death during follow-up in those with ventricular arrhythmia. But there is also a relationship between the presence of arrhythmia and cardiac death not occurring suddenly, suggesting that ventricular arrhythmias relate to the severity of disease within the heart, the extent of the latter being the important determinant of survival. Indeed, further studies have confirmed the association between the presence of advanced grades of ventricular extrasystoles and the degree of left ventricular impairment[28]. The relationship can be extended further (similar findings have been noted with exercise testing) in that the severity of ventricular arrhythmia is related to the severity of coronary arterial disease[29]. Interestingly, in a study examining both the grade of arrhythmia and ejection fraction, sudden death occurred in those with low ejection fractions and arrhythmias of low grade[30].

Angiographic studies, on a population who had been resuscitated from ventricular fibrillation but who had prior myocardial infarction, demonstrated that the vast majority had extensive left ventricular impairment and stenosis of at least two major coronary arteries[31]. It might, therefore, not be regarded as surprising that no study has yet managed to demonstrate that control of ventricular extrasystoles by drugs can prevent sudden death. The studies using antiarrhythmic drugs in the post-infarction period undertaken prior to the CAST (Cardiac Arrhythmia Suppression Trial) study were criticized on various grounds. In many of the trials, there was no requirement for an arrhythmia to be present for patients to be enrolled into the study. The trials, furthermore, involved single drugs and there was no opportunity for either the dose to be tailored to the need of the individual, nor for another drug to be substituted if the first drug was unsuitable. The studies did not require that the drug suppressed the ventricular extrasystoles, and none was large enough to detect a significant reduction in mortality[32].

The CAST study was undertaken in the knowledge that asymptomatic ventricular extrasystoles were a risk factor for death after myocardial infarction, and that physicians, particularly in the USA, often treated these arrhythmias. The trial was well designed to test the hypothesis that suppression of ventricular extrasystoles by one of three antiarrhythmic agents would reduce the rate of death. In addition to the converse being shown, namely, that both encainide and flecainide increased the mortality compared to the group receiving the placebo, the study revealed an unexpectedly low rate of mortality for the placebo group[13]. This may have, in part, reflected the high level of care and supervision of the patients in the study, but it also reflected the recruitment of patients with low levels of ventricular arrhythmia, many of whom were entered more than a year after their episode of infarction. The increased mortality as a consequence of therapy with either encainide or flecainide is a further example of proarrhythmic activity. This effect was notable in the CAST studies for persisting throughout the trial, whereas previous experience with proarrhythmic effects has suggested that the risk was limited mostly to the period immediately after the start of treatment. This may well represent the additional interaction between antiarrhythmic drugs, their proarrhythmic action, and a population prone to recurrences of ischaemia.

Even if the grade of ventricular arrhythmia (extrasystoles, couplets and so on) revealed by ambulatory monitoring is important, the arrhythmic event immediately leading to sudden cardiac death is ventricular fibrillation with or without antecedent rapid ventricular tachycardia. There is an inherent limitation in treating ventricular extrasystoles on the basis that they trigger the lethal ventricular arrhythmia, particularly if the treatment, as in the CAST study, only attempts to eradicate a percentage, albeit 80%, of the ventricular extrasystoles. An additional hypothesis, namely that the marker arrhythmia will respond in an individual patient in the same way as the target arrhythmia may also be erroneous. It has been shown that treatment of a marker present on ambulatory monitoring may well differ in pharmacological responsiveness when compared with the major target[33].

There have, therefore, been alternative approaches based on an attempt to define directly the degree of electrical instability of the ventricular myocardium. This approach has been generated by the development of programmed electrical stimulation for the study of supraventricular and ventricular tachycardia. Study of patients with ventricular tachycardia has defined stimulation protocols as necessary for induction of clinical arrhythmias. These protocols have been applied prospectively to populations of patients recovering from myocardial infarction in an attempt to define the group at risk of sudden death.

Initial studies concentrated on the repetitive ventricular response (a non-stimulated ventricular extrasystole after a single ventricular extrastimulus introduced during atrial pacing) as an index of ventricular electrical instability and demonstrated that it predicted occurrence of both ventricular tachycardia and sudden death after myocardial infarction[34]. Subsequent studies[35,36] questioned the validity of this relationship. More recent approaches have used more vigorous protocols of stimulation in an attempt to discriminate those patients at high as opposed to low risk. The results obtained so far, however, are conflicting. Deniss et al.[37] demonstrated that the combination of programmed stimulation and exercise testing predicted virtually all deaths occurring within the first year after myocardial infarction, as well as identifying, when both tests were negative, a population with an excellent prognosis in the first year. Roy et al.[38], in contrast, failed to identify a group at high risk when using programmed stimulation, although both sudden death and the occurrence of spontaneous ventricular tachycardia were predicted by the findings of a low ejection fraction, ventricular aneurysm, and exercise-induced ventricular extrasystoles. Interestingly, the rates of inducibility of ventricular arrhythmia in the two studies were similar, suggesting that differences in protocols used for stimulation and in the numbers of patients receiving beta-blockers were not relevant. Further evaluation will be necessary on these, and similar methods of assessing electrical instability, before their value is established as routine investigations.

These studies have revealed the presence, in a subset of patients after myocardial infarction, of the substrate for sustained ventricular arrhythmia. As the mechanism of ventricular tachycardia in the majority of those with ischaemic heart disease has been shown to be re-entry, and that disordered intramyocardial conduction is known to be an essential prerequisite[39], other techniques have been employed in order to identify patients with abnormally slowed conduction. The areas involved are small and the resultant delayed electrograms of microvolt amplitude. Standard electrocardiographic techniques are not capable of registering these signals, but they can be detected by high gain amplification and signal averaging[40]. Such delayed electrograms (late potentials) appear after the end of normal ventricular depolarization and are almost ubiquitous in those with coronary arterial disease complicated by spontaneous ventricular tachycardia[41]. They are also present in many who have not had sustained ventricular tachycardia and are not present in many of those who have been resuscitated from ventricular fibrillation. For the present, the recording of a signal averaged electrocardiogram is routinely used by few centres, although it may prove a useful screening test to identify those at increased risk for future arrhythmic events. It is, therefore, worthy of further investigation[42].

Ventricular tachycardia

The distinction between patients who die suddenly as a result of a lethal ventricular arrhythmia and those who present with sustained ventricular tachycardia is narrow. It seems likely that the electrical characteristics of a spontaneously occurring arrhythmia determine the haemodynamic response, although susceptibility to ischaemia may also be relevant. In a comparison of patients with aborted sudden death and those with sustained ventricular tachycardia, Stephenson et al.[43] noted a faster rate of induced tachycardia at electrophysiological study, and noted multiple sites of infarction in those with the 'lethal' form of arrhythmia. These findings correlated with a higher incidence of syncope during induced tachycardia in the group undergoing aborted sudden death. They agree with another study[44] which noted the importance of the cycle length of tachycardia as a major determinant of syncope during tachycardia. These data suggest that modification of the induced cycle length of the tachycardia by antiarrhythmic drugs may prevent the tendency for rapid rates to degenerate into fibrillation, such evidence being suggested by a study which suggested an improved survival when the rate of induced tachycardia was slowed by more than 100 ms, especially by amiodarone[45].

The absence of direct evidence that antiarrhythmic therapy improves prognosis in patients with ventricular arrhythmia remains a tantalizing hurdle. Clinical observation indicates that ventricular tachycardia is associated with sudden death, and that antiarrhythmic drugs can prevent the tachycardia, but there is no evidence from studies of populations that the prognosis is improved as a consequence of the antiarrhythmic therapy[46]. This discrepancy may, in part, be explained by the tendency of antiarrhythmic drugs also to have proarrhythmic actions, with the end result that those who benefit from the drugs are balanced by those who suffer the ill consequences. It remains to be seen whether newer techniques of treatment, such as surgical resection or electrical techniques based on the implantable defibrillator will demonstrate similar drawbacks. Uncontrolled data following implantation of defibrillators suggests that their subsequent rates of survival exceed those which could be expected with antiarrhythmic drugs and, possibly, with surgery[47].

Electrophysiological studies in survivors of sudden cardiac death

The increasing success of cardiopulmonary resuscitation inititated by bystanders and prehospital defibrillation, and the increasing numbers of patients able to leave hospital, has revealed the high recurrence rate for future events in those whose arrest did not occur in the context of acute myocardial infarction. Follow-up studies have shown recurrence of cardiac arrest in 10–30% during the first year after discharge from hospital[8,9,17]. Various interventions have been proposed in an attempt to reduce mortality due to further cardiac arrest but the optimal method of assessing therapeutic efficacy is still debatable.

Programmed electrical stimulation has been assessed in a number of studies. In a significant number, although lower than in those presenting with sustained ventricular tachycardia, sustained ventricular arrhythmias can be induced[8,10,18,33,48]. The rates of non-inducibility vary between 20% and 40%. In general, those who are non-inducible have better ventricular function and less severe coronary arterial disease than those in whom arrhythmias can be induced. Rates of survival have shown that inducibility, and more severe ventricular dysfunction, are associated with a worse prognosis. Patients with preserved left ventricular dysfunction in whom arrhythmias cannot be induced appear to have a good outlook without specific antiarrhythmic therapy, especially if other features such as ischaemia are treated.

In those with inducible ventricular arrhythmia, either sustained ventricular tachycardia or ventricular fibrillation, this endpoint has been used to assess therapeutic interventions designed to render the patient non-inducible and, thereby, to identify those with an improved prognosis. Various studies have demonstrated an improved survival in those who became non-inducible with either antiarrhythmic drugs or antiarrhythmic surgery. A recent investigation of the largest population yet to be studied, however, has published differing results[49]. There was no improved survival in those whose inducible arrhythmia could be suppressed by therapy, and no difference between those with inducible ventricular tachycardia or ventricular fibrillation. Further studies will be required to determine whether differences in the protocol of stimulation or the definition of a non-sustained arrhythmia contributed to these discrepancies. It seems certain that programmed stimulation has a different role in the assessment of cardiac arrest compared with those with sustained ventricular tachycardia. Non-inducibility at baseline in the presence of poor left ventricular function indicates a poor outlook. Implantation of a defibrillator may then be the only therapeutic option. Further methods to stratify the risk in those in whom it is possible to induce a ventricular arrhythmia remain a priority.

References

1. Adgey, A.A.J., Nelson, P.G., Scott, M.E., et al. Management of ventricular fibrillation outside hospital. Lancet, i, 1169, 1969
2. Pantridge, J.F. and Adgey, A.A.J. Pre-hospital coronary care: the mobile coronary care unit. Am. J. Cardiol., 24, 666–673, 1969
3. Baum, R.S., Alvarez, H. and Cobb, L.A. Mechanisms of out-of-hospital sudden cardiac death and their prognostic significance. Circulation, 48 (Suppl. 4), 40, 1973
4. Alvarez, H., Wills, R.E. and Cobb, L.A. Sudden cardiac death: physiologic boservations and therapeutic implications. Am. J. Cardiol., 31, 116, 1973
5. Cobb, L.A., Conn, R.D. and Samson, W.E. Prehospital coronary care: the role of a rapid response mobile intensive coronary care system. Circulation, 43 (Suppl. 2), 139, 1971
6. Liberthson, R.R., Nagel, E.L., Hirschman, J.C. and Nussenfeld, S.R. Prehospt ventricular defibrillation. Prognosis and follow-up course. N. Engl. J. Med., 291, 317–321, 1988
7. Goldstein, S., Landis, J.R., Leighton, R., et al. Characteristics of the resuscitated out-of-hospital cardiac arrest victim with coronary heart disease. Circulation, 70, 538–546, 1984
8. Myerburg, R.J., Kessler, K.M., Estes, D., et al. Long-term survival after prehospital cardiac arrest: analysis of outcome during an 8 year study. Circulation, 70, 539–546, 1984
9. Schaffer, W.A. and Cobb, L.A. Recurrent ventricular fibrillation and modes of death in survivors of out of hospital ventricular fibrillation. N. Engl. J. Med., 293, 260–265, 1975
10. Wilber, D.J., Garan, H., Finkelstein, D., et al. Out-of-hospital cardiac arrest. Use of electrophysiologic testing in the prediction of long-term outcome. N. Engl. J. Med., 318, 19–24, 1977
11. Report of the Joint International Society and Federation of Cardiology/World Health Organisation Task Force on Standardization of Clinical Nomenclature. Nomenclature and criteria for diagnosis of ischaemic heart disease. Circulation, 59, 607–609, 1979
12. Greene, H.L., Richardson, D.W., Barker, A.H., et al. Classification of deaths after myocardial infarction as arrhythmic or non-arrhythmic (The Cardiac Arrhythmia Pilot Study). Am. J. Cardiol., 63, 1–6, 1989

13. Cardiac Arrhythmia Suppression Trial (CAST) Investigators. Prelimary Report: Effect of encainide and flecainide on mortality in a randomized trial of arrhythmia suppression after myocardial infarction. *N. Engl. J. Med.*, **321**, 406–412, 1989
14. Reichenbach, L.D., Moss, N.S. and Meyer, E. Pathology of the heart in sudden cardiac death. *Am. J. Cardiol.*, **39**, 765–772, 1977
15. Davies, J.M. Pathological view of sudden cardiac death. *Br. Heart J.*, **45**, 88–96, 1981
16. Warnes, C.A. and Roberts, W.C. Sudden coronary death: relation of amount and distribution of coronary narrowing at necropsy to previous symptoms of myocardial ischaemia, left ventricular scarring and heart weight. *Am. J. Cardiol.*, **54**, 65–70, 1984
17. Cobb, L.A., Baum, R.S., Alvarez, H.A. and Shaffer, W.A. Resuscitation from out of hospital ventricular fibrillation: four years follow-up. *Circulation*, **51,52 (Suppl. III)**, 223–228, 1975
18. Myerberg, R.J., Conde, C.A., Sung, R.J., *et al*. Prehospital cardiac arrest: early and longterm clinical and electrophysiological characteristics. In *Sudden Death* (eds H.E. Kulbertus and H.J.J. Wellens), Martinus Nijhof, Thee Hague, pp. 219–231, 1980
19. Lawrie, D.M., Higgins, M.R., Godman, M.J., *et al*. Ventricular fibrillation complicating acute myocardial infarction. *Lancet*, **ii**, 523–528, 1968
20. Vismara, L.A., DeMaria, A.N., Hughes, J.L., *et al*. Evaluation of arrhythmias in the late hospital phase of acute myocardial infarction compared to coronary care unit ectopy. *Br. Med. J.*, **37**, 598–603, 1975
21. Julian, D.G. and Campbell, R.W.F. Sudden death. In *Scientific Foundations of Cardiology* (eds P. Sleight and J. Van Jones), William Heineman, London, pp. 220–223, 1983
22. Campbell, R.W.F., Murray, A. and Julian, D.G. Ventricular arrhythmias in the first 12 hours of acute myocardial infarction: National history study. *Br. Heart J.*, **46**, 351–356, 1981
23. Lie, K.I., Wellens, J.H., VanCapelle, F.J. and Durrer, D. Lidocaine in the prevention of primary ventricular fibrillation. *N. Engl. J. Med.*, **291**, 1324–1329, 1974
24. Noneman, J.W. and Roger, J.F. Lidocaine prophylaxis in acute myocardial infarction. *Medicine*, **57**, 501–515, 1978
25. May, C.S., Furberg, C.D., Eberlein, K.A., *et al*. Secondary prevention after myocardial infarction. A review of short-term acute phase trials. *Prog. Cardiovasc. Dis.*, **25**, 335–360, 1983
26. Koster, R.W. and Dunning, A.J. Intramuscular lidocaine for prevention of lethal arrhythmias in the prehospitalisation phase of acute myocardial infarction. *N. Engl. J. Med.*, **313**, 1105–1110, 1985
27. Ruberman, W., Weinblatt, E., Goldberg, J.D., *et al*. Ventricular premature complexes and sudden death after myocardial infarction. *Circulation*, **64**, 297–302, 1981
28. Bigger, J.T., Fleiss, J.L., Kleiger, R., *et al*. The Multicenter Postinfarction Research Group. The relationship among ventricular arrhythmias, left ventricular dysfunction and mortality in the 2 years after myocardial infarction. *Circulation*, **69**, 250, 1984
29. Bruce, R.A., De Rouen, T., Peterson, D.R., *et al*. Noninvasive predictors of sudden cardiac death in men with coronary heart disease. Predictive value of maximal stress testing. *Am. J. Cardiol.*, **39**, 833–840, 1977
30. Schultze, R.A., Strauss, H.W. and Pitt, B. (1977). Sudden death in the year following myocardial infarction. *Am. J. Med.*, **62**, 192–197, 1977
31. Weaver, W.D., Lorch, G.S., Alvarez, H.A. and Cobb, L.A. Angiographic findings and prognostic indicators in patients resuscitated from sudden death. *Circulation*, **54**, 895–900, 1976
32. Fuberg, C.D. Effect of antiarrhythmic drugs on mortality after myocardial infarction. *Am. J. Cardiol.*, **52**, 32C–36C, 1983
33. Myerberg, R.J., Conde, C., Sheps, D.S., *et al*. Antiarrhythmic drug therapy in survivors of prehospital cardiac arrest: Comparison of effects on chronic ventricular arrhythmias and recurrent cardiac arrest. *Circulation*, **59**, 855–863, 1979
34. Greene, H.L., Reid, P.R. and Schaeffer, A.H. The repetitive ventricular response in man. An index of ventricular electrical instability (abstract). *Am. J. Cardiol.*, **41**, 400–405, 1978
35. Mason, J.W. Repetitive beating after single ventricular extrastimuli: incidence and prognostic significance in patients with recurrent ventricular tachycardia. *Am. J. Cardiol.*, **45**, 1126–1131, 1980
36. Farshidi, A., Michelson, E.L., Greenspan, A.M., *et al*. Repetitive responses to ventricular extrastimuli: incidence, mechanism and significance. *Am. Heart J.*, **100**, 59–68, 1980
37. Denniss, A.R., Baaijens, H., Cody, D.V., *et al*. Value of programmed stimulation and exercise testing in predicting one-year mortality after acute myocardial infarction. *Am. J. Cardiol.*, **56**, 213–220, 1985
38. Roy, D., Marchand, E., Theroux, P., *et al*. Programmed ventricular stimulation in survivors of an acute myocardial infarction. *Circulation*, **3**, 487–494, 1985
39. Josephson, M.E., Horowitz, L.N., Farshidi, A., *et al*. Sustained ventricular tachycardia; evidence for protected localized reentry. *Am. J. Cardiol.*, **42**, 416–424, 1987

40. Simson, M.B. Identification of patients with ventricular tachycardia after myocardial infarction from signals in the terminal QRS complex. *Circulation*, **64**, 235–242, 1981
41. Breithardt, G. and Borggrefe, M. Recent advances in the identification of patients at risk of ventricular tachyarrhythmias; role of ventricular late potentials. *Circulation*, **85**, 1091–1096, 1987
42. Cripps, T.R., Bennett, E.D., Camm, A.J. and Ward, D.E. Inducibility of sustained monomorphic ventricular tachycardia as a prognostic indicator in survivors of recent myocardial infarction: A prospective evaluation in relation to other variables. *J. Am. Coll. Cardiol.*, **14**, 289–296, 1989
43. Stevenson, W.G., Brugada, P., Waldecker, B., *et al.* Clinical, angiographic and electrophysiologic findings in patients with sustained ventricular tachycardia after myocardial infarction. *Circulation*, **6**, 1146–1152, 1985
44. Hamer, A.W.F., Rubin, S.A., Peter, T. and Mandel, W.J. Factors that predict syncope during ventricular tachycardia in patients. *Am. Heart J.*, **107**, 997–1002, 1984
45. Waller, T.J., Kay, H.R., Spielman, S.R., *et al.* Reduction in sudden death and total mortality by antiarrhythmic drug testing: criteria of efficacy in patients with sustained ventricular tachyrrhymia. *J. Am. Coll. Cardiol.*, **10**, 83–89, 1987
46. Swerdlow, C.D., Winkle, R.A. and Mason, J.W. Determinants of survival in patients with ventricular tachyarrhythmias. *N. Engl. J. Med.*, **308**, 1436–1442, 1983
47. Gabry, M.D., Bradman, R., Johnston, D., *et al.* Automatic implantable cardioverter–defibrillator: patient survival, battery longevity and shock delivery analysis. *J. Am. Coll. Cardiol.*, **9**, 1349–1356, 1987
48. Roy, D., Waxman, H.L., Kienzle, M.G., *et al.* Clinical characteristics and long-term follow-up in 119 survivors of out-of-hospital cardiac arrest: relation to inducibility at electrophysiologic testing. *Am. J. Cardiol.*, **52**, 969–974, 1983
49. Poole, J.E., Mathisen, T.L., Kudenchuk, P.J., *et al.* Long-term outcome in patients who survive out of hospital ventricular fibrillation and undergo electrophysiologic studies: evaluation by electrophysiologic subgroups. *J. Am. Coll. Cardiol.*, **16**, 657–665, 1990

Index